MW00561203

Heal Your Shoulder at Home (and Get Results!)

Heal Your Shoulder at Home (and Get Results!)

Self-treatment rehab guide for shoulder pain from frozen shoulder, bursitis and other rotator cuff issues

ISBN 978-0-9971626-7-7

The authors gratefully acknowledge the contributions of the following persons:

Legal advice by Charles L. Thoeming, ASCENDANT (R) Legal Services, ASCENDANT IP (R), Lafayette, California
Cover design and advice by Molly Williams, Big Hat Press, Lafayette, California
Anatomical drawings by Rose Wright Design, Walnut Creek, California
Professional photography by Jeff Kay Smith, Walnut Creek, California
(with some ad hoc photos by the authors)

Medical Disclaimer:

Before starting the treatment program presented in this book, it is imperative that you get the advice of a qualified medical professional to confirm that you are in good enough health to pursue these exercises and that they are suitable for your particular condition. Listen to your body, and if any of the exercises in this book cause undue discomfort, then please discontinue the exercises. Consult with your practitioner as needed for guidance. Use this book at your own risk.

Contents

Introduction

Who this book is for

This book is suitable for anyone who has been told by their doctor that they need to do shoulder stretching and strengthening exercises. Some of the most common conditions to which this applies include arthritis, bursitis, tendonitis, and adhesive capsulitis (frozen shoulder). If you haven't already, be sure to get a medical examination before putting this book into practice.

Why another shoulder book?

We have noticed a variance between how shoulder conditions are commonly treated versus a great many other medical conditions. It's hard to visit a doctor these days and not get some physical parameter measured and recorded in your chart as a *number*; for example, your height, weight and blood pressure are very likely to be recorded. Other data points might include your temperature, cholesterol, blood sugar level, bone density, visual acuity, etc. On the other hand, if you see a doctor about shoulder pain she will probably take your arm and bend it this way and that, but no measurements will be taken and no numbers recorded. An x-ray may also be taken and perhaps an injection of cortisone to reduce inflammation. If no major problems show up on the x-ray, you may be given a list of exercises to do at home and sent on your way. This may be a good start, but shoulder pain is usually associated with reduced range of motion (ROM) which needs to be improved before returning to normal activities; otherwise, there is a distinct possibility of reinjury. But how do you know how much progress you're making, and if you've improved enough to consider the treatment as complete? In this book we give you criteria for when to consider your shoulder well again, and ***ways to measure your progress along the way***. We also present the standard at-home treatments and exercises that you can use on your own to get well.

Making Shoulder Therapy More Quantitative

In this book we treat healing your shoulder as a project. First, we recommend that you **assess your current status** by measuring your range of motion in **both** shoulders. A physical therapist can do this and we also give you ways of doing it yourself. Based on that, you can **set goals** as to what you want to accomplish with your treatments. For example, you might want to recover the same range of motion in your weak shoulder that you have in your well shoulder. In order to reach your goals you **make a plan** which might involve such things as hot and cold compresses, and stretching and strengthening exercises. As you execute the plan, you can **monitor your progress** and **make adjustments** as necessary. In addition, you can also **make forecasts** as to when your treatment might be completed. For this to be most effective, your progress needs to be expressed numerically.

In support of the above, we advocate measuring the **distances** of several core stretching exercises. This is not typically done, but doing this enables the patient to be much more consistent in the exercises and also makes progress vastly more visible. We find that being able to readily see the results of one's efforts is very motivational. It helps the patient to go from being passive to proactive, helpless to confident, pessimistic to optimistic. Knowledge is power, and empowering you to take charge of your condition is what this book is all about.

How to Use This Book

We suggest that you read straight through chapters 1 through 12 first, but omit chapters 9 and 11. Chapters 9 and 11 give step by step directions for doing various exercises and aren't needed until you actually start to do them. The other chapters give a lot of information on *why* we are doing the exercises and general information on *how* to do them, which will make your performance of the exercises much more effective.

After that, please feel free to start doing the exercises that you and your medical practitioner agree would be most beneficial. You can also re-read various sections and visit the Appendixes as your needs evolve.

Some Conventions Used In This Book

For brevity and consistency, we call the shoulder you are doing therapy on your "weak" shoulder. The arm on that side is called your "weak" arm and that hand your "weak" hand. Your other shoulder we call your "well" shoulder and so forth.

We refer to *range of motion* a lot in this book. We will usually abbreviate it as ROM.

When referring to hypothetical patients, rather than writing "he or she," we just write "she." We think that's logical since more women suffer from shoulder problems than men.

To address your shoulder issue you might see a variety of medical professionals such as general practitioners, orthopedic surgeons, physical therapists and others. Unless the topic at hand calls for distinguishing between the various types of medical professionals, we will usually just refer to them all as "practitioners," or possibly as "she" as appropriate to the context.

We do repeat ourselves a bit in this book. There are two reasons for this: one is that we don't expect all readers to retain everything from just one reading. And two is that we expect readers to jump around a lot in this book, so we want to improve the odds that they get exposed to our main points.

Who is the "We" in This Book?

Although the copyright shows a single author, Melvin Rosenthal, the narration of the book is in the first person plural, "we." This reflects the involvement of the author's wife, June, without whose input this book wouldn't have been written. June sewed the prototype therapy straps, tested the exercises, read the first draft, and provided the motivation to develop these ideas into something that could be shared with other people. Therefore, we thought that "we" is appropriate.

Equipment Needed

We recommend the following seven types of equipment for your therapy, although you could get by with less if necessary. We give a ball-park estimate for the price of each type of equipment and estimate that the whole set would cost around $197 plus any shipping and tax. However, some of this you may already have such as hot and cold packs, a pole, weights and/or bands, and a strap that could be used for stretching. For many of these items, it's possible to use substitutions, such as a soup can or other heavy object instead of the bands and weights. Other items can be improvised. If cost is a critical factor, then equipment costs can be brought down to zero. If you have this book in your possession, then you have everything you need to get started.

The two items unique to our therapy method are the blocks and the strap. (We also refer to them as "therapy blocks" and "therapy straps.") We sell these items, but you can also improvise if you need too. The strap is similar to the commonly-used yoga straps, but for our use, it needs to have a scale in inches imprinted on it similar to a tape measure used in sewing. A stack of books and magazines can also be substituted for the blocks, saving $76, although the blocks, with their standard sizes, *are* a convenience. All of these items are discussed in greater detail in Appendix 4, including suggestions as to where to acquire them or how to improvise them.

Item	Cost
Bands, elastic, for strengthening exercises (2)	$11
Blocks, for stretching and measuring	$76
A cane, rod, or pole to aid in stretches	0
Hot/cold packs (2)	$12
Pulley, for stretching	$10
Strap, for stretching and measuring	$28
Weights, for strengthening exercises	$60

Part One:

Getting Started

1—I Have a Sore Shoulder, Now What?

First, STOP all activities that led to your shoulder pain. The first mistake that many people make is to try and go on as before in the hopes that the problem will go away in a short time and without any treatment. They take a pain killer and proceed as though nothing has happened, or they go from playing tennis three times a week to only twice a week. That might work for a sore muscle, but it won't work for an injured shoulder. You probably have inflammation and this needs to be reduced for the pain to go away and healing to start. Your shoulder tissue also has minimal blood flow, especially in the tendons, so it may take months or even years for it to heal. If you don't treat your injury properly, it may never fully heal.

Second, if you haven't seen a doctor yet, do so. There are many conditions that affect the shoulder such as arthritis, bursitis, tendonitis, adhesive capsulitis, rotator cuff tears, impingement, and thoracic outlet syndrome to name a few. *You need a diagnosis and guidance that you are ready to do stretching and strengthening exercises before proceeding with this program.*

Third, don't treat your condition as an isolated incident that you will heal from and then return to business as usual. It may never again be "business as usual." Why is that? Because once you've injured your shoulder, the possibility of reinjury is greater—one source says that 27% of sports injuries are actually reinjuries[1]. And if you injure your shoulder a second time, then a third injury will be even more likely.

However, depending on your injury, this downward spiral doesn't have to be inevitable. Many people who injure their shoulder won't rehabilitate it properly and take the steps necessary to keep it in good shape, but you can—it's your choice. Through the knowledge available in this book, and proper flexibility and strengthening exercises, it's possible that some people will be able to emerge from therapy with a shoulder that's more flexible and stronger than it was before their injury.

Fourth, be aware that we naturally lose flexibility in our shoulders as we age, perhaps as much as 25 percent[2]. Many experts consider flexibility to be one of the key elements of fitness along with such things as endurance, strength, core strength, and balance[3]. When we injure our shoulders we often lose some of that flexibility—it can be as if we've aged decades in just one day! The main goal of many shoulder treatments is to fight back and regain as much of that flexibility as possible. Why? Because shoulder flexibility is critical for much of our work, play, and daily living. Think of the careers that require flexibility such as painter, plumber, carpenter, mechanic or nurse. Think of the recreation we do that employs our shoulders such as golf, tennis, baseball, gardening, and dancing. Consider the Activities of Daily Living that use our shoulders such as combing our hair, bathing, and dressing. If we have restricted range of motion (ROM) we are liable to reinjure our shoulder just by doing these normal activities so that we end up back in the doctor's office again for treatment. However, that scenario isn't inevitable. For many people, they can maintain their youthful flexibility well into old age if they're willing to work at it. Now let's get started.

2—Treatment Overview

The "Twelve-Step" Program

1. Assess your current status and set goals. You should have a diagnosis of what your shoulder problem is from your doctor and a general plan as to how to treat it. We recommend that you get your range of motion in both shoulders measured in degrees as soon as possible in your treatment. A physical therapist can do this and perhaps other practitioners as well. You will typically have to ask that this be done as it is not routine. However, as you read through this book, hopefully we will convince you that insisting on this is worth the trouble. Chapter three lists six different shoulder movements that we like to have measured. The reason for having it measured in degrees is that there are guidelines established for what constitutes healthy ROM and they are expressed in degrees. We presume you'd like to be within the guidelines for ROM, just as you'd like to be within the guidelines for your weight, blood pressure, cholesterol and so forth.

In addition to measurements in degrees, you will also be measuring your ROM in terms of distances as you do the stretching exercises in this book. This is built into our key exercises so that you will always know what progress you are making regardless of any other measurements that you or your practitioner might take.

You can then set goals and work with your practitioner to manage your rehabilitation. Chapter three delves deeper into this process.

2. Improve your posture. Many people don't realize it, but slouching can compress the shoulder capsule putting pressure on the tissue inside and causing premature wear and tear[4]. Therefore, this is something you can do RIGHT NOW—even as you're reading this—to give you a head start on healing your shoulder. This is discussed further in Chapter 4.

3. Water. On WebMD there's a slideshow titled "7 Wonders of Water".[5] One of the "wonders" is that water helps lubricate our joints. Obviously, a well-lubricated shoulder is easier to move. Conversely, a dehydrated shoulder would be stiffer and more painful to move; so we might want to drink a little extra water, even if we don't feel thirsty. What we like to do is be aware of the time, and every hour or so make sure we have water close at hand and have a few extra sips.

4. Aerobic exercise. If you haven't been doing aerobic exercises lately, now might be a good time to start. The Mayo Clinic tells us that aerobic exercise helps to prevent heart disease, high blood pressure, stroke, type 2 diabetes, obesity, colds, and flu (by boosting the immune system) and even cancer.[6] If that's not reason enough, it also boosts our mood and prompts the body to release hormones called endorphins which are natural pain killers. A reduction in pain helps us to stretch further when doing our ROM exercises, and a boost in mood gives us more energy to help us do our therapy on a regular basis.

It's best to use the aerobic exercise as an opportunity to get hydrated by drinking water before, during, and after the exercise. If possible, it's very effective to follow the aerobic exercise with a hot shower and then with the stretching routines. The heat and hydration from the aerobics and shower provide the optimal preparation for getting the absolute best benefit from our stretching exercises.

5. Hot and cold treatments. Cold *reduces* blood flow to your shoulder relieving swelling, inflammation and pain. On the other hand, heat *increases* blood flow to the shoulder which helps healing. It also relaxes our tissue and allows us to do our exercises more effectively and with less likelihood of further injury.

6. Medications. Your doctor may prescribe pills or injections. It must be remembered that these are *not* a *cure*, but only a means of reducing inflammation, swelling, and pain so that you can do your shoulder treatments more effectively. Medications also have side effects and so should only be taken on the advice of a medical practitioner. Keep in mind that aerobic exercise and icing also address the same problems as meds do, but without the side effects.

7. Stretching exercises. While the tissue in our shoulder is healing, we start stretching exercises. As much as possible, we try to prevent our shoulder from stiffening up further, and we start to loosen it up if we can. This can help prevent frozen shoulder as well as reinjuries.

8. Strengthening exercises. We lose ROM in our shoulders because of stiffness, muscle weakness, and pain. If we stop using our shoulders because of an injury, our muscle strength can decrease up to 17 percent within the initial 72 hours, so it's good to start some mild strengthening exercises as soon as we can safely do so.[7]

9. Winding down. Once we've reached our ROM goals, we don't just abruptly stop doing our exercises; if we do, there's a good chance that our shoulder will start to stiffen up again. For this reason, we gradually taper off from our exercises. For example, we might go from stretching twice a day, to once a day, to every other day, to three times a week, etc.

10. Final healing. Your shoulder pain may go away before your shoulder is completely healed. Don't risk reinjury by resuming activities prematurely. Consider giving your shoulder a few more weeks to heal even after the pain stops.

11. Resuming activities. Remember from chapter 1 that once we've had a shoulder injury, we're more likely to experience a reinjury, perhaps 27% or so. In order to avoid that scenario, we want to ease back into any activities that might aggravate the shoulder. For example, if you're goal is to play tennis three times a week, you might start with once a week for two weeks, then twice a week for two weeks before trying for three times a week.

You would also want to constantly monitor for any signs of pain or returning stiffness and immediately cease the activity if these should occur. Only after you've become pain-free and your ROM is on target should you try again to gradually return to your activity.

12. Maintenance. Avoid doing things that might hurt your shoulders. Monitor your shoulders periodically to check for any pain or reduced ROM. Continue with some stretching and strength training as needed to stay in tip top shape.

Sample Weekly Routine

Below is a sample weekly workout routine to illustrate how the major pieces discussed in this chapter might fit together. It is made up of five elements: hot and cold treatments, stretching, aerobic exercise, and strength training. Of course, we couldn't begin to tell people how they should put their own schedule together since there are just too many unknowns, but the sample does illustrate some basic principles. It's always good to apply some sort of heat before stretching, whether a hot pack or a hot shower. It's always good to stretch twice a day, even if one of the sessions is brief, since our muscle memory is very short and we rapidly digress if we don't keep at it. We take advantage of the aerobic exercise by doing it before any stretching as another way of warming up. And finally, icing is done last to reduce any inflammation or pain that has built up during the day.

How much extra time will your shoulder therapy take? Hopefully, not much if you can multitask. The hot and cold treatments can be done while you're watching TV or eating, etc. Perhaps the stretching and strength training can be done while the evening news is on. You take showers anyway, and possibly you're already doing aerobics, so this may not take any extra time. By taking charge of your therapy and working diligently on your own you may be able to get by with fewer trips to your practitioner which will save you travel time and costs in the long run.

SAMPLE WEEKLY ROUTINE						
Mon	**Tue**	**Wed**	**Thurs**	**Fri**	**Sat**	**Sun**
Morning						
heat	heat	heat	heat	heat	heat	heat
stretch	stretch	stretch	stretch	stretch	stretch	stretch
Afternoon						
aerobic	heat	aerobic	heat	aerobic	heat	heat
shower	stretch	shower	stretch	shower	stretch	stretch
stretch	strength	stretch	strength	stretch	strength	ice
ice	ice	ice	ice	ice	ice	

3—Managing Your Recovery

Assessing Your Current Range of Motion

If you don't know where you're starting from or where you're going to, then it's hard to plan the trip; so the first thing we want to know is where you're starting from with regards to your range of motion. There are six key movements that we are most interested in. The table gives the name of each movement, a brief description of each, as well as guidelines for minimum desired ROM for each movement. In case you find the descriptions hard to follow, you can see illustrations of them in chapter 9. For the movements below, we describe the movements from a standing position, although in chapter 9 the patient lies down to perform them (except for "reach behind the back").

Key range of motion movements

Movement	Minimum ROM	Full ROM
1. Flexion	120°	180°

Raise your arm up in ***front*** of you towards the ceiling. Your arm at your side is zero degrees and straight up is 180 degrees.

2. Abduction	120°	180°

Raise your arm straight out to the ***side*** towards the ceiling.

3. Horizontal External Rotation	65°	90°

Hold your arm horizontally straight out to the side, then bend at your elbow to make a right angle with your forearm pointed straight out in front of you. This is zero degrees. Now rotate your forearm upwards towards the ceiling. Straight up is 90 degrees.

Movement	Minimum ROM	Full ROM
4. **Horizontal Ext Rot at Side**	65°	90°

Keep your arm down at your side, then bend at the elbow to make a right angle with your forearm pointed straight out in front of you. This is zero degrees. Now rotate your arm towards your back. Straight out from your side would be 90 degrees.

5. Horizontal Internal Rotation	60°	75°

Hold your arm horizontally straight out from your side, bend at your elbow to make a right angle in the horizontal plane. This is zero degrees. Rotate your forearm down towards the floor. Straight down would be 90 degrees.

6. Reach behind the back	70°	115°

Your arm straight down at your side is zero degrees. Make a fist. If you can place your knuckles in the small of your back, then you have moved your forearm up approximately 70 degrees. If you can reach the tips of your fingers to the bottom of your opposite shoulder blade, that would make about a 115 degree angle from the floor. These measurements are the most inexact of the six due to individual differences in body build. In this case, *where* you can place your hand behind your back is more significant than the degrees measurement.

As we stated previously, you can ask a physical therapist to give you measurements in degrees for the movements listed above for both of your shoulders. She or he is likely to wonder why you want both shoulders measured. Usually, patients don't ask for measurements, let alone for both shoulders. Hopefully, it would be sufficient to explain that you want to get the readings for both shoulders so that you can see how much ROM you've lost in your weak shoulder so that you can get an idea of how far you have to go in your recovery.

Another option is to measure your ROM on your own with an instrument called a *goniometer*. Appendix 7, Resources, gives a source where you can buy these instruments. Appendix 7 also describes what to search for on Google to bring up YouTube videos that explain how to use the device.

Setting Goals

Once you have these measurements, you can set your goals. Your initial goal might be to get the ROM in your weak shoulder equal to that in your well shoulder. If that turns out to be unobtainable, then you might just try to get all of your ROMs up to the suggested minimums as given in the table above.

Simpler Ways of Assessment and Goal Setting

Your ROM doesn't have to be measured in degrees. At home we find it easier to measure it in inches. For example, stand facing a wall and with the hand of your well shoulder reach up as far as you can and make a pencil mark at that point. Then, reach up with your other hand as far as you can and make another pencil mark. (If you actually do this, you might want to stick painter's tape to the wall and make your marks on that.) You could then use a tape measure to determine how far you can reach with each hand. That is a measure of your *flexion.* Your goal for flexion might simply be to close the gap so that you have the same ability with your weak arm as with your well arm. We have ways of measuring the stretch for all six of the movements given in the table and it involves no extra work—it's an integral part of doing the exercises. The important thing is to avoid just spinning your wheels—we want to make *progress*.

Logging Your Progress

In the chart that follows is an example of how we record our progress. This example is for *static lying flexion*. (See Chapter 9 for illustrations of what it looks like.) In this exercise the patient starts out by lying down with her weak arm at her side. (Note that the model is a "he," but we are continuing with our convention of referring to the patients as "her.") She then raises her arm up towards the ceiling and back down towards the floor until it comes to rest as close to the floor as possible. In this example, the weak shoulder is the right one. Initially, the patient can lift that arm up in a 130 degree arc as opposed to the well arm which she can lift 170 degrees. This assumes that she was able to get a measurement in degrees of her movement in this direction; otherwise, just the recording in inches would do. (The inches measurement would simply be the distance from her hand to the floor when she has fully extended her arm.) She has set as her goal that she wants her right shoulder to be as flexible as her left shoulder. Note that stretches are not being done with the left arm; a measurement was taken for that arm to keep as a benchmark, and for comparison with her right arm. The patient is stretching her right arm once and holding the stretch for 30 seconds.

Stretching Log: <u>Static Lying Flexion</u>

	Left					Right			
Date	Degrees	Inches	Reps	Time		Deg.	Inches	Reps	Time
05/14/17	170	4.00	1	30		130	13.50	1	30
05/15/17							13.50		
05/16/17							13.50		
05/17/17							13.50		
05/18/17							13.25		
05/19/17							13.25		
05/20/17							13.25		
05/21/17							13.25		
05/22/17							13.00		
05/23/17							13.00		
05/24/17							13.00		
05/25/17							12.75		
05/26/17							12.75		
05/27/17							12.75		
05/28/17							12.50		

Appendix 5 provides a blank worksheet which you can copy to record YOUR progress.

Forecasting Major Milestones and Treatment Completion Date

In order to forecast when we might complete our recovery and be able to resume our normal activities, we focus on three major phases of the healing process: stretching, strength building, and winding down/final healing.

From the table in the previous section we can see that it took the patient about two weeks to gain one inch in flexion. She wants to get down to four inches from the floor which is eight and a half inches from where she is now. We can calculate that at one inch every two weeks it will take her about 17 more weeks to get to where she wants to be. Similar logs and calculations can be done for the other five key ROM movements. The furthest-out completion date for all six of the key movements will mark the completion of the stretching phase of recovery.

We can do a similar procedure for our strength building program. In the sample on the next page, we've picked out five exercises that all strengthen the rotator cuff muscles. (For a description of what the rotator cuff is, see Appendix 1.) This is an illustration only, as you and your practitioner might select different exercises and different goals for each exercise.

In the sample Forecast Worksheet on the next page, the patient started doing her strength training midway through her stretching program. She was winding down the stretching program while the strength training was building up. After she met her strengthening goals, she started to taper off of both the stretching and strength building for one month. She then gave her shoulder a final two weeks to heal before starting to gradually resume her normal activities. She also made a commitment to follow the maintenance program described in chapter 12 to prevent her shoulder problem from recurring.

Forecast Worksheet **Prepared 10/01/17**

STRETCHING	START	FINISH
Static Lying Flexion	05/14/17	09/24/17
Horizontal external rotation at side	05/14/17	08/15/17
Horizontal external rotation	05/14/17	10/15/17
Horizontal internal rotation	05/14/17	07/14/17
Abduction	05/14/17	10/01/17
Internal rotation behind the back	05/14/17	10/05/17
STRENGTH TRAINING		
Internal rotation	08/01/17	10/15/17
External rotation	08/01/17	10/15/17
Scaption	09/01/17	12/04/17
Seated dumbbell horizontal external rotation	09/01/17	11/03/17
Standing diagonal dumbbell raise	09/01/17	12/01/17
WINDING DOWN/FINAL HEALING	12/02/17	01/15/18

In addition to being handy for your own planning purposes, completing an initial forecast of your treatment program and then updating it periodically is useful for communicating your status to other people. A great many people are unaware of how long it can take to recover from a shoulder problem. If it takes more than a month for your shoulder to heal you may hear such things as "Are you still having a problem with your shoulder? Why is it taking so long to get better? Can't they operate on it?" On this latter point, hopefully you have a clear understanding with your practitioner as to why or why not an operation was or wasn't performed. In terms of the length of the recovery time, when you're armed with your systematically-developed forecast, you can now start to educate people. You can tell them that it takes a long time to stretch tissues and strengthen muscles, but that you're 40% through with your program and you expect to resume your activities at the first of the year or whenever it might be.

Appendix 3 gives a blank forecast worksheet which you are free to copy for your own use, or three columns drawn onto some lined paper would work fine, too.

Making Adjustments to Stay on Track

If for any reason you're not satisfied with the progress you're making, such as how long it's taking or the amount of range of motion that you're recovering, there may be some things you can do to produce better results:

- Make sure you do your stretching exercises *every* day with no exceptions for birthdays, holidays, travel, minor illnesses, etc. This is because your shoulder has limited "memory" and will tend to return to its original shape after 24 hours, the same way that a rubber band returns to its original shape.[8] Do the strengthening exercises faithfully, too, of course.
- If you're currently doing your exercise session once per day, then increase it to twice per day, or whatever your practitioner recommends. You might at least do *some* of the exercises twice per day.
- Do a wide variety of stretching and strengthening exercises. There is a synergy effect: gains in one area will facilitate gains in other areas as well.
- Prepare for your exercises better by doing the following: Do aerobic exercises before stretching, build up a sweat and drink a pint of water so that your shoulder is lubricated, then, take a good hot shower.
- Increase the number of times you go to physical therapy to as many as three times per week.
- Take advantage of the buddy system. Let someone know that you're doing shoulder therapy and have them check up on you to make sure that you're doing your exercises regularly. They could even observe you doing the exercises and make sure that you're doing them correctly. This can be a win/win situation as it strengthens your relationship while you strengthen your shoulder.

Case Study

The case study which follows shows how a shoulder problem may evolve over time and is probably typical for many people. It illustrates the importance of seeking qualified medical help and following their instructions, as well as employing the suggestions presented in this book.

The subject of the study was a female, age 83. In approximately August of 2015 she began to experience pain in her right shoulder. Since the pain was fairly mild, she continued with her daily activities, hoping that the pain would go away on its own. Her daily activities were fairly ordinary, but she did like to go square dancing and ballroom dancing each week which involved a lot of arm movement, such as under-arm turns. The pain didn't go away, and on December 22, 2015, she went to see her general practitioner about it. The problem was diagnosed as bursitis, an inflammation of the bursa. (The bursa is a sack of fluid in your shoulder which allows the muscles, tendon and bones to slide smoothly past one another.) An injection of cortisone was administered to reduce the inflammation, and the patient was sent home with a list of shoulder stretching and strengthening exercises to do. After three days, the shoulder pain was completely gone and the subject felt that she was cured. For this reason, she never bothered to do the exercises.

However, by June of 2016, the pain returned. By October of that year she concluded that the pain was not going to go away on its own and sought the advice of the author of this book, Melvin Rosenthal. Melvin took a set of ROM measurements for both of her shoulders which can be seen in Appendix 2 as the first set of bar graphs dated 10/13/16. What was immediately obvious was that she had less ROM in her right shoulder than in her left shoulder in all six of the movements tested. Another observation was that movement behind her back for the right arm was quite painful and restricted and didn't meet guidelines. Lastly, although her flexion ability was within guidelines, it wasn't adequate for the lifestyle that she was leading. For the dancing she needed to be able to raise her right arm almost straight up over her head, which she was unable to do. We believe that the stress of trying to do this motion, given her reduced ROM, was probably a major cause of her problem and may have been the reason why the bursitis lingered on and on.

The patient immediately started doing the stretching exercises found in this book. A full set of exercises was done once a day, preceded by a heat treatment before and a cold treatment afterwards. For a while she still continued with her dancing, but at the beginning of February, 2017, she ceased dancing altogether. By this time there was improvement in all of her ROM movements. However, although her shoulder pain was reduced, some still remained. On February 16, 2017, the patient visited her MD to confirm her progress and see if she was on track for recovery. The doctor gave her another cortisone shot to try and reduce the residual pain.

Again, the pain went away in about three days, but she still continued to refrain from dancing, and did continue with her stretching exercises. On March 16th she visited a physical therapist for an evaluation who noted that she still had some stiffness in her abduction movement. Therefore, she continued her stretching exercises until the end of March. The results at that time are shown in the graphs in Appendix 2 dated March 28, 2017. She was pain-free and had adequate ROM in all her movements, so she resumed her dancing as of April third. She also started shoulder strength training at that time which she will continue indefinitely. For the first month she monitored her ROM weekly, then switched to monthly. She checks daily for any signs of pain. If there are any signs of problems, she will immediately take remedial actions.

Some observations and lessons learned:

- The patient took no remedial steps to treat her symptoms for months after their onset. She should have seen her doctor within a week of the onset of the problem.
- She should have stopped dancing immediately when the pain occurred and cut back on everything else that might irritate her shoulder.
- She should have begun ice treatments at home for two days after the onset of symptoms, then begun heat treatments.

- After her first doctor visit, she should have done the exercises that were prescribed.
- Injections are not a cure; you have to be both pain-free and have adequate ROM and strength to suit your lifestyle before resuming activities.
- If professional help is required, then consult with BOTH your primary care practitioner and a physical therapist. The PT can fine-tune your exercises to ensure that adequate ROM is achieved.
- The stretching exercises WORK. The patient eventually achieved better ROM in her weak arm than in her well arm for behind-the-back movements and horizontal internal rotation.
- Be informed and proactive. Shoulder rehabilitation requires doing stretching exercises *every day*, and you need to know how to do them properly. Ask questions. Study this book. Get measurements of your ROM in BOTH shoulders at the start of your treatment.

4—Improve Your Posture

"Practicing proper posture will reduce issues in all parts of the body, from head to toe." Dr. Karl Knopf

We all know that poor posture can strain the back, but it can also contribute to shoulder problems as well.[9] What is good posture?

When standing, pretend that there is a string attached to the top of your head and pulling you straight up. Your ears, shoulders, hips and ankles should all be in a straight vertical line. Pull your belly in. Don't lock your knees, and keep your weight mostly on the balls of your feet. To test your posture, stand against a wall pressing your bottom, shoulder blades, and head against the wall while keeping your heels about two to four inches away from the wall. There should be just enough space to slide your hand in the curve behind your back (your lumbar curve). If not, adjust the space by tightening your abdominal muscles to decrease it or arch your back to increase it.

When sitting, you should have a chair which allows your feet to rest comfortably on the floor with your upper legs parallel to the floor. A footrest may be used if desired. Your ankles should rest just in front of your knees and don't cross your knees. Your back should have support in the lumbar curve area. If your chair doesn't provide this, consider going to a medical supply store and trying out back rests to use with your chair, or maybe even spring for a good new chair if you spend a lot of time sitting. Even a small pillow, cushion, or rolled towel in the small of your back would be better than nothing. Sit up straight with your head over your shoulders and your shoulders relaxed in a neutral position.

For more information on posture, the Mayo Clinic has a good write-up, including illustrations. See Appendix 7, "Selected Resources."

5—Natural Remedies: Cold, Heat, Aerobic Exercise, and Water

Cold and heat treatments deliver a one-two punch of healing to your shoulder. Cold reduces swelling in your shoulder which allows blood to flow more freely, while heat draws blood into your shoulder which promotes healing.

Although Ice treatments initially *reduce* the flow of blood to your shoulder, they relieve swelling, inflammation, and pain which ultimately allows for greater blood flow. Ice your shoulder as soon as possible after an injury. You can use ice from your fridge or a cooling pack from the drug store or other sources. To avoid freezing the skin, don't place the cooling medium directly against the skin—there should be at least a thin layer of cloth between the two. Ice may be applied for ten to 15 minutes, but no more than that to avoid damaging skin and nerves. Also, stop if the skin becomes numb. Employ the cold treatments for 24 to 48 hours after an injury.

Heat treatments *increase* the flow of blood to your shoulder muscles and tendons. Since they have a limited number of blood vessels, this extra stimulation can really aid in healing. Some ways of applying heat include a hot water bottle, a heating pad set to low, moist hot towels, a hot shower, or hot packs available from the drug store that you heat in the microwave. Moist heat is the best. Be careful not to burn your skin and limit heating time to ten to 15 minutes.

After the initial use of ice to treat an injury, there is no universally agreed upon formula for the best ways to use heat and cold for your shoulder. It's mostly a matter of trial and error along with advice from your medical practitioner. Sometimes, mostly heat seems to work best; sometimes, mostly cold; and sometimes, alternating the two. Whatever you do, a quick cool-down after exercising can't hurt and may help to reduce any inflammation and pain.

Aerobic exercise and drinking lots of water are effective ways of preparing your shoulder to get the most out of your stretching exercises. Drinking a pint of water while working out hard enough to produce a mild sweat will lubricate your shoulder allowing for freer ROM. The heat buildup through aerobics also relaxes the muscles allowing them to stretch further. Finally, aerobic exercise produces hormones, called endorphins, which reduce your pain threshold and again allow you to stretch further. If the aerobic exercise is followed by a brief hot shower, that also helps to relax the shoulder and get the blood flowing.

6—Medications

This chapter describes a few common medications and is included primarily for reference. It may answer some questions that you might have, or make you better informed when discussing the pros and cons of medications with your doctor. It is NOT to be taken as a recommendation from the authors to take any drugs on your own. Please discuss with your practitioner whether drugs are right for you. Many more drug descriptions can be found on the website Drugs.com.

We wish to emphasize here that ***even if our shoulder is pain free, it doesn't always mean that our shoulder is healthy and fit.***[10] For example, if a doctor has us take pills or gives us a cortisone injection, our pain may subside, but in many cases we will still be left with reduced range of motion and strength. In order to be fit for work, play, and other activities, we need to make sure that those issues are addressed. Therefore, the bottom line is don't ease back into your activities until you have been given the all-clear from your practitioner.

Non-Steroidal Anti-Inflammatories (NSAIDS)

Generic Name: Ibuprofen.
Some Brand Names: Advil, Motrin.
What it is: A non-steroidal anti-inflammatory drug.
Benefits: It reduces hormones that cause inflammation and pain.
Some possible side effects: May increase risk of heart attack and stroke. Can cause stomach and intestinal bleeding. May exacerbate asthma, liver and kidney disease in people who have those conditions.

Generic name: Naproxen.
Some Brand Names: Aleve, Midol Extended Relief.
What it is: A non-steroidal anti-inflammatory drug.
Benefits: It reduces hormones that cause inflammation and pain.
Some possible side effects: The same as for Ibuprofen.

Steroids

Generic Name: Cortisone
What it is: Cortisone is a steroid made by the adrenal gland. It is released to counteract stress. The cortisone used in shots is a synthetic that resembles natural cortisone but is more potent and longer lasting (up to several weeks).

Benefits: Cortisone is a powerful anti-inflammatory that is often used to treat bursitis and tendonitis—two common conditions that affect the shoulder. Cortisone injections are more powerful than NSAIDS taken orally because they deliver a relatively large amount of medication directly to the affected site.

Some possible side effects: One side effect is a "cortisone flare." This occurs when the injected cortisone crystallizes and can cause significant pain for a day or two. Another possible side effect is an infection, especially if the injection is made into a joint, as it commonly is. Cortisone can also cause weakening of cartilage and tendons. For this reason, some doctors limit the frequency of cortisone injections and may put a limit on the number of injections they give for a particular problem.

Generic Name: Dexamethasone
Some brand names: Decadron, Dexamethasone Intensol, Dexasone, Hexadrol.
What it is: Dexamethasone is another form of steroid. It is taken orally for such things as arthritis, blood/hormone/immune system disorders, allergic reactions, certain skin and eye conditions, and others.

Benefits: The same as for other steroids, but taking it orally has some advantages: the doctor doesn't have to hit the exact spot as with injections, it's not painful like an injection may be, and the dosage may be spread out over a number of days or weeks rather than all at once.
Some possible side effects: Stomach upset, headache, dizziness, trouble sleeping, weight gain, and menstrual changes.

Part Two:

Stretching Exercises

7—Why Stretch?

To Prevent Adhesive Capsulitis, "Frozen Shoulder"

When our shoulder is sore, the natural tendency is to want to avoid pain and protect it by keeping it as immobile as possible. For example, if we have a broken arm, we put it in a cast and don't move it at all so that it can heal properly. However, in the vast majority of cases, with a sore shoulder our best bet is to do the exact opposite by keeping it moving by doing stretching exercises and mild strengthening exercises. Why? One reason is to avoid adhesive capsulitis, commonly known as frozen shoulder, which can set in very quickly if we don't move our shoulder. With adhesive capsulitis lesions form between the shoulder capsule and the top of our upper arm bone (the *humerus*) which makes movement difficult. Frozen shoulder is quite painful, debilitating, and can last for years, so we certainly want to avoid it. If we already have it, we need to do these exercises to regain as much of our range of motion as we can, which brings us to our second reason for stretching...

To regain Range of Motion (ROM)

Range of motion is essential for performing the activities of daily living such as bathing, grooming, and dressing. Although our shoulder pain usually resolves itself eventually on its own without treatment, unless we do stretching exercises, we may not regain as much ROM as we had before our injury.

To prevent reinjury

If our shoulder motion is restricted, we may reinjure our shoulders simply by trying to do the same activities that we're used to doing every day such as lifting a child, reaching overhead for a suitcase, or swinging a tennis racket.

To improve self esteem

If you end up with permanently restricted ROM in one shoulder, your body won't be symmetrical; you'll feel lopsided, and this is uncomfortable. Also, as we've said, we all lose flexibility as we age; keeping as much of our flexibility as we can helps us to feel younger.

8—How to Stretch Effectively

Similarity to Strength Training

For most of our stretching exercises we use a similar method as we use in strength training. In strength training we move our limbs in a certain way, a set number of times, against a ***resistance*** measured in ***pounds*** (or kilograms). We start at a resistance that is safe and comfortable and move upwards from there.

In our stretching exercises, we move our arms in a certain way, a set number of times, through a ***distance*** measured in ***inches*** (or centimeters, for our metric friends). Likewise, we start at a distance that is safe and reasonably comfortable and increase it from there.

However, keep in mind that stretching should be done every day, while strength training for shoulder rehabilitation should be done two or three times per week.

Getting the Most from Your Stretching

People often don't get the benefit they should from stretching for three main reasons:

ONE is that they don't stretch vigorously enough and thus make minimal progress. We solve this problem by trying to have the distance of each stretch be equal to or greater than in our previous session. Thus, we always try to go forward in our range of motion, never backwards.

However, we must always let pain be our guide; for example, one exception to the rule might be if we have adhesive capsulitis. This condition has three phases: *painful/freezing, frozen,* and *thawing*. The painful phase is just that—if we move our arm suddenly or much outside our comfort zone, we feel severe pain. In the first two stages our ROM becomes more and more restricted so that we may reluctantly go backwards in our stretching exercises. In the thawing phase, the pain gradually subsides and we regain some or all of our ROM. With diligent stretching, we may be able to regain more of our ROM than we would otherwise, and also possibly shorten our recovery time.

TWO is that they push themselves too hard and suffer more pain and are forced to ease off of the exercises. To avoid this, you can rate your discomfort in doing the exercises on a scale of 1 to 10 and never go above a 2. We also ease slowly into the stretch, hold the stretch, then ease off gently; we never "bounce." It's also a good idea, especially at the beginning of your treatments, to have an experienced professional such as a physical therapist work with you as you do the exercises to make sure you have the correct form and that you don't overdo it.

We also put limits on how fast we try to progress. We suggest a few simple rules which will become clearer when we go into the exercises in detail:

- We only increase our stretching distances in increments of 1/4 of an inch at a time. Stretch each distance at least two days in a row. After four days in a row, see if you can increase a stretch by the fifth day.
- Never stretch more than an inch beyond where gravity alone pulls your arm.
- Never increase your stretch in more than two exercises on the same day.

THREE is that patients don't do the exercises every day. After stretching, your tissues immediately start to go back to their previous length, and after about 24 hours, you may have given up most of your gains.[11] Therefore, in order to make steady progress, it's best to stretch every day and maybe even twice a day. Our hope is that as you increase your stretches and see the progress that you're making that you'll be motivated to do the exercises regularly. Maybe you'll even look forward to your workouts with enthusiasm!

Passive versus Active Stretching

Passive stretching. These exercises are those where your weak shoulder muscles don't have to do any work to do the stretch. An example of this would be an examination by your doctor where the doctor takes your arm with both of her hands and moves it herself to test your ROM. Another example would be for your well arm to lift up your weak arm using a rope passing through an overhead pulley (this is a common exercise).

Active stretching. These exercises are those where the muscles of your weak shoulder do all of the work to move the shoulder through its ROM. An example of this would be moving your weak arm unassisted over your head, such as with our door jamb exercise.

Active Assistive. This is a blend of the two previous modes of stretching. For example, while moving our weak arm up a door jamb we could grasp the weak arm at the elbow with our well hand, and push up a little with our well arm to gently assist our weaker arm.

With this classification scheme you can match the exercises to the current level of recovery of your shoulder and thus make better progress while reducing the chances of further injury. As you might expect, the passive exercises are the easiest to do. Therefore, as we start our treatments, we start out with the easiest (passive) and work our way up to the most difficult (active). If doing an exercise gets to be more than two on the pain scale, then you might try using the other arm to assist to make it easier. If this doesn't work, then simply stop doing the exercise and try it again later when your shoulder has recovered more.

Dynamic versus Static Stretching

Static stretches. With this stretch you move your arm to a certain position and hold it in place for a *relatively* long period of time compared to dynamic stretching. We recommend a stretch time of 30 seconds. If you can't hold the stretch for 30 seconds without significant pain, then don't stretch quite so far. We only do each static stretch one time; i.e., one repetition.

Dynamic stretches. These involve much more movement. We typically stretch 10 to 15 times, but we only hold the stretch for a second or two. The advantage to dynamic stretches are that they increase blood flow to the shoulder and hence healing, and they also warm the shoulder up which allows the muscles to stretch further and reduces the risk of injury.

Aim to do both types of stretches slowly and smoothly. There should be no bouncing or rocking motions. That type of motion can cause further injury.

Stretching Routines

Our preferred program for stretching is to do it twice a day—a short session in the morning, and a longer session in the afternoon or evening. This keeps you constantly stretched out and avoids the stiffening that occurs after 24 hours. In the morning session you regain some or all of the ROM that you may have lost overnight. You don't have to do all of the exercises, just enough to get limbered up a bit. A suggested routine is below. The morning session need not be long, either—ten minutes or so will do—although you can make it longer if you wish. We don't try and progress in the morning session; that is, we don't try and stretch any further in any of the exercises; we leave that for the afternoon session. It's also not necessary to record what we've done in the morning session.

The afternoon/evening session is where we make the most progress. This starts with good preparation: get well hydrated beforehand, consider doing some aerobic exercise to build up a sweat, and maybe take a shower. Then, do a full program of stretches and see if you can increase your stretching distance in any of the stretches. One way to do that is to do a stretch the same distance as the previous time. If that seems easy and there is no pain, then increase the distance by 1/4 inch and try it again. If that goes well, then that is your new benchmark for that exercise. During this session, you will need to record the stretches that you have done using the log form. The six static stretches listed in **bold** are the key ones that stretch us in six different ways and can be measured, so they should be recorded. The pulley and wall reach exercises are also easy to measure and it doesn't hurt to keep track of them, either. Note that we don't try and measure or keep track of the dynamic stretches. We just go by feel for those.

Finally, everybody is different so please feel free to adjust this program if some other schedule would suit you better. For example, if you're a morning person and really exercise better in the morning, then you might want to make that your main session for the day. Likewise, if you have a really demanding job and are just exhausted at the end of the day, you might want to do your stretching before work rather than after. Do what works for you.

Sample Morning Stretching Routine

1. Optional aerobic workout

2. External Heat if no aerobic exercise was done

A hot shower is best; alternatively, use a hot pack or pad for up to 15 minutes.

3. Dynamic Stretches—Do each up to ten times

- Pendulums
- Shoulder Box
- Lying Horizontal Abduction/Adduction (a.k.a. lateral drops)
- Dynamic Lying Flexion
- Standing Internal Rotation With Rod (Back Scratch)

4. Static Stretches—Do each one once for 30 seconds

- **Static Lying Flexion**
- **Horizontal External Rotation at Side**
- **Horizontal External Rotation**
- **Horizontal Internal Rotation**
- **Abduction (Angels)**
- **Standing Internal Rotation With Strap (If not too painful)**

Sample Evening Stretching Routine

1. Aerobic exercise if part of your routine

2. External Heat

A hot shower is best; alternatively, use a hot pack or pad for up to 15 minutes.

3. Dynamic Stretches—Do each one up to ten times

- Pendulums
- Shoulder Box
- Elbow Touches
- Lying Press
- Lying Horizontal Side to Side
- Dynamic Lying Flexion
- Standing Extension With Rod (Reverse Lift)
- Standing Internal Rotation With Rod (Back Scratch)

4. Static Stretches—Do each one once for 30 seconds

Bold type denotes the key stretches that you should record on your log forms.

- **Static Lying Flexion**
- **Horizontal External Rotation at Side**
- **Horizontal External Rotation**
- **Horizontal Internal Rotation**
- Pulley Stretch
- **Abduction (Angels)**
- **Standing Internal Rotation With Webbing**
- Wall Reach

5. Cool Down—Ice for up to 15 minutes

9—Stretching Exercises

Pendulums

Purpose: Warm up and loosen the shoulder to get the most from other exercises and to prevent injuries.

Directions

- There are three ways of doing these exercises: forward and back, side to side, and around in circles. Mix it up on different days if you like.
- Using your well arm, lean over and brace yourself on a solid object and dangle the weak arm.
- Swing your arm forward and back.
- Swing your arm side to side.
- Swing your arm around in circles; clockwise, then counter clockwise.
- Start doing these exercises passively by using body sway to get your arm swinging. As you progress in your recovery, you can use your shoulder muscles to assist in the motion. You can also try grasping a one-pound dumbbell to give your arm more momentum in the swings.

Lean over, dangle your weak arm, and do the pendulum exercises of your choice.

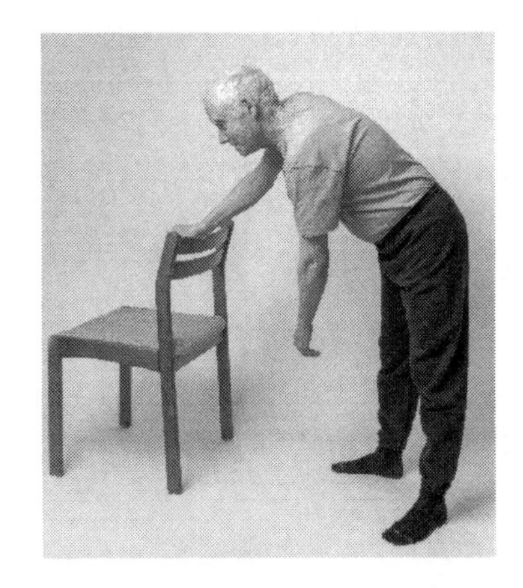

Shoulder Box

Purpose: Warm up and loosen up the shoulder.

Directions

- Stand up straight with good posture, arms at sides.
- Lift your shoulders straight up (shrug your shoulders).
- Roll your shoulders back, bringing your shoulder blades towards each other, and chest out.
- Lower your shoulders, then return to neutral starting position. Repeat 10X.
- When you get used to this you can do it in more of a continuous flowing motion, and perhaps do five forward then five backward.

1-Start

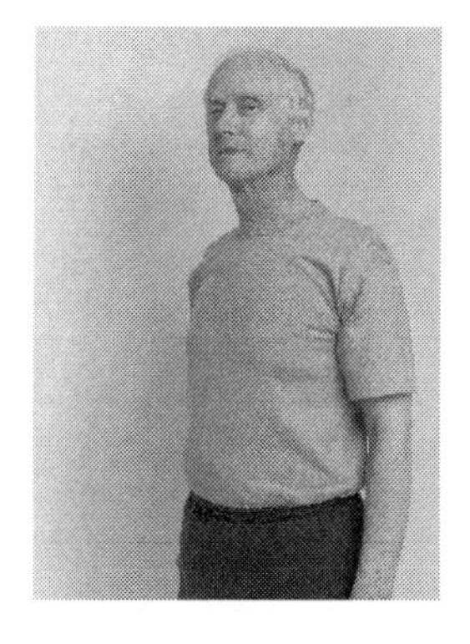

2-Up

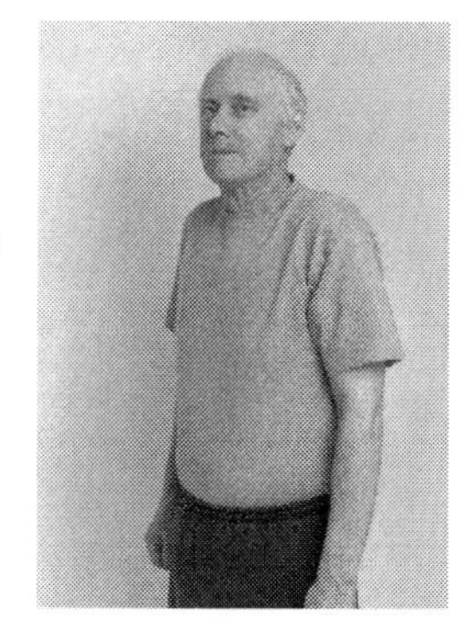

3-Back

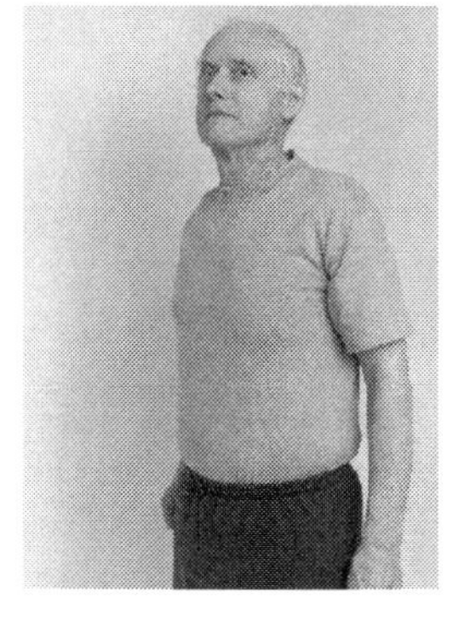

4-Down, then back to start

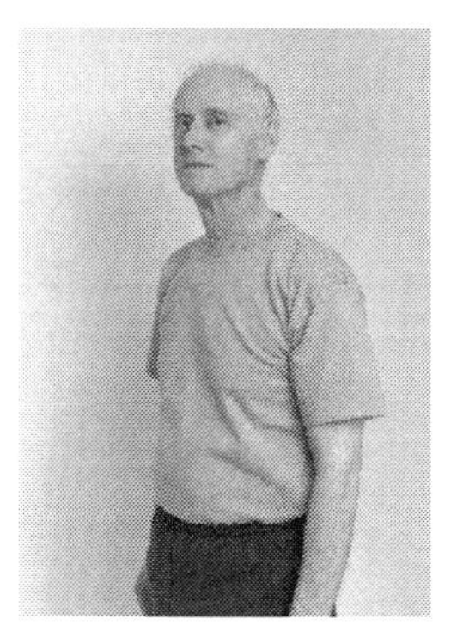

Elbow Touches

Purpose: Provides a warm up and mild stretch of the shoulder.

Directions

- Sit or stand with good posture.
- Start with hands behind neck and fingertips touching, elbows out at 45 degree angle.
- Bring your elbows together as far as you can without any pain.
- Move elbows out to the side while squeezing your shoulder blades together.
- Repeat together and apart movements several times.

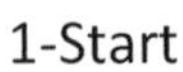
1-Start

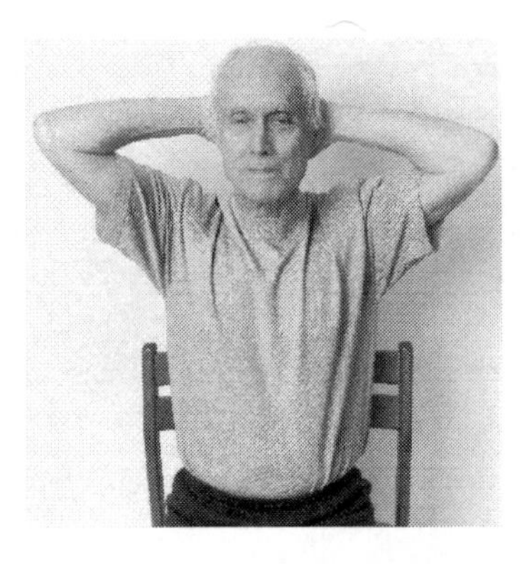

2-Elbows Together

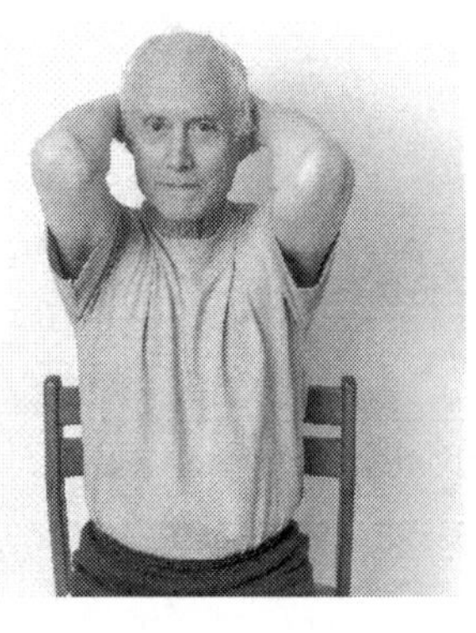

3-Elbows Apart

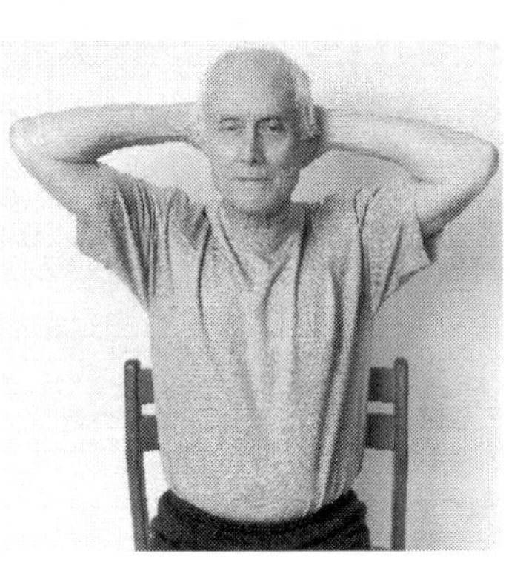

Lying Press

Purpose: Warm up, mild stretch and strength building, and preparation for flexion exercises.

Equipment Needed: A cane, stick or rod about 2-1/2 feet long. Pictured is a window curtain "projection rod."

Directions

- Lie on your back with knees bent for comfort.
- Hold rod in both hands, elbows on floor close to your sides, forearms pointed upwards.
- Slowly press the rod up towards the ceiling until arms are straight.
- Slowly bring the arms down to starting position and repeat up to ten times.

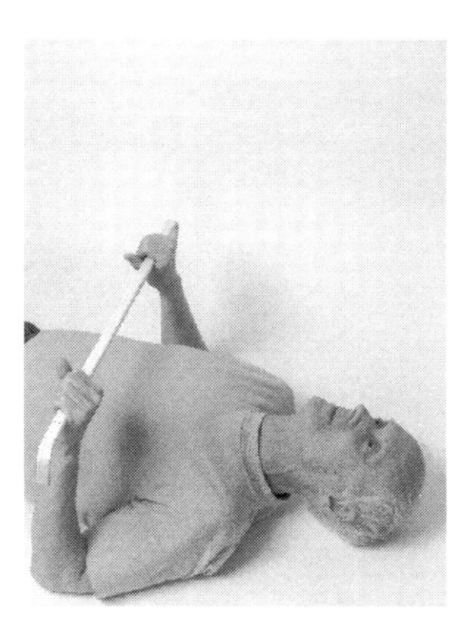

Start

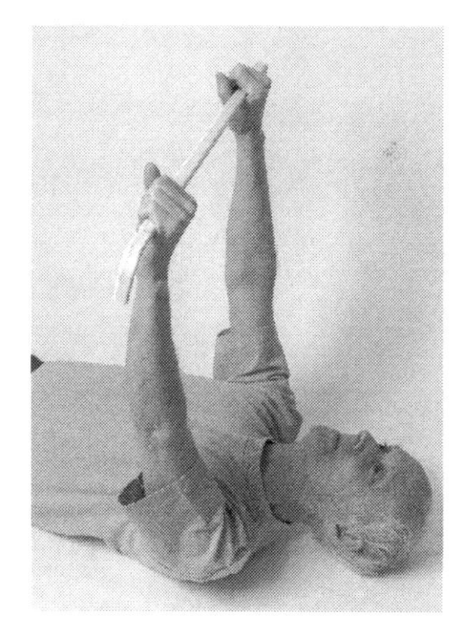

End

Horizontal Side-to-Side with Cane

Purpose: Increase side-to-side range of motion. This exercise is also known as "Horizontal Abduction/Adduction" or "Lateral Drops." Different authors may call the same exercise by different names—they're not standardized.

Equipment Needed: Cane or rod of some sort.

Directions

- Lie on your back with knees bent for comfort.
- Hold rod in both hands with your arms extended straight up and your shoulder blades slightly drawn together.
- Slowly move your arms to the right as far as you can without pain, keeping both shoulders on the floor.
- Hold the stretch for about two seconds then return to starting position.
- Repeat the stretch to the left. Do up to ten times.

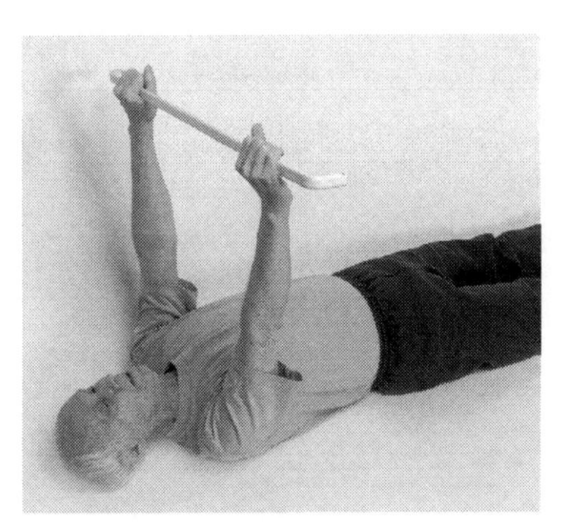

Start

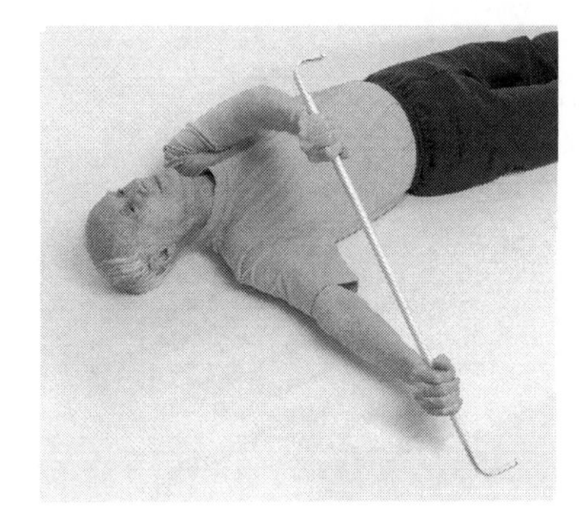

Stretch right & left

Dynamic Lying Flexion

Purpose: Warm up flexion exercise.

Equipment Needed: Cane or rod of some sort.

Directions

- Lie on your back with knees bent for comfort.
- Hold rod in both hands with your arms extended straight up and your shoulder blades slightly drawn together.
- Slowly move the rod up and over your head and down towards the floor as far as you can without pain.
- Hold the stretch for a second or two then return to starting position.
- Repeat up to ten times.

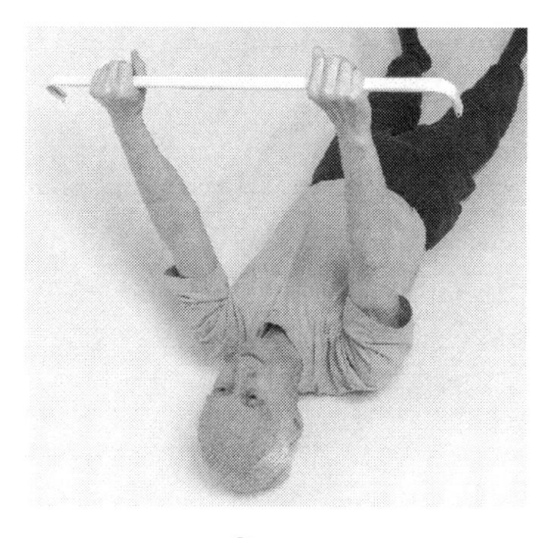

Start

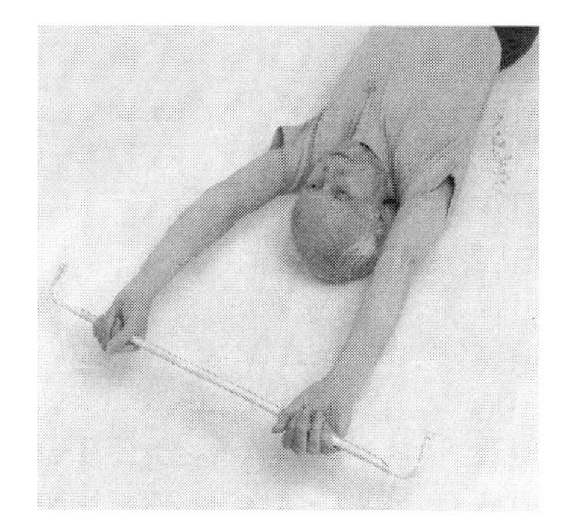

End

Standing Extension with Rod (a.k.a. "Reverse Lift")

Purpose: Good starting exercise to improve ability to reach behind the back. This helps in putting on a belt, tucking a shirt in, or reaching for a back pocket.

Equipment Needed: Cane, stick, or rod of some sort.

Directions

- Stand up straight with good posture.
- Hold a rod behind your back with your hands about shoulder width apart and your palms facing backwards.
- Slowly extend the rod backwards, keeping your arm straight. Be careful not to overdo it.
- Hold the stretch for a second or two then return to starting position.
- Repeat up to ten times.
- As your ability in this movement improves, try moving your hands closer together as you do it. Eventually, you may be able to do it with your hands touching. One way to do this is to wrap two strips of painter's tape around the rod about 14 inches apart and grasp the rod at the tape. Every fifth day try moving the strips an inch or two closer together.
-

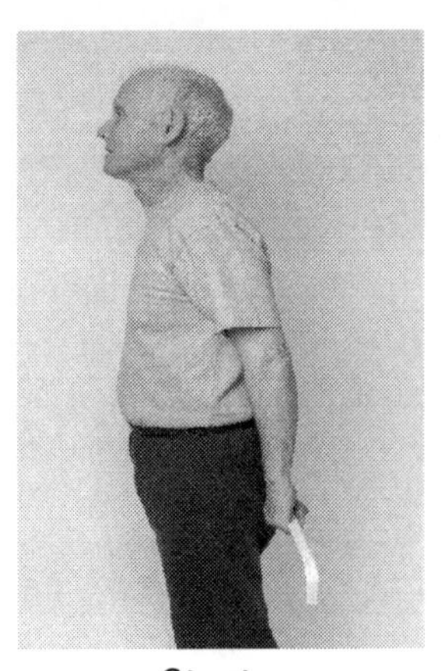
Start

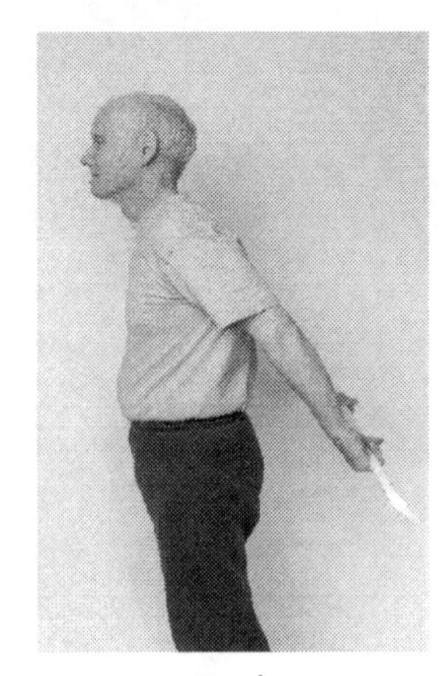
End

Standing Internal Rotation with Rod

(a.k.a. "back scratch")

Purpose: Increase ability to do movements behind the back.

Equipment Needed: Cane, stick, or rod of some sort.

Directions

- Stand up straight with good posture.
- Hold a rod behind your back with your hands about shoulder width apart and your palms facing backwards.
- Slowly lift the rod up behind your back as high as you comfortably can.
- Hold the stretch for a second or two then return to starting position.
- Repeat up to ten times.
- As your ability in this movement improves, try moving your hands closer together as you do the movement. Eventually you may be able to do it with your hands touching.

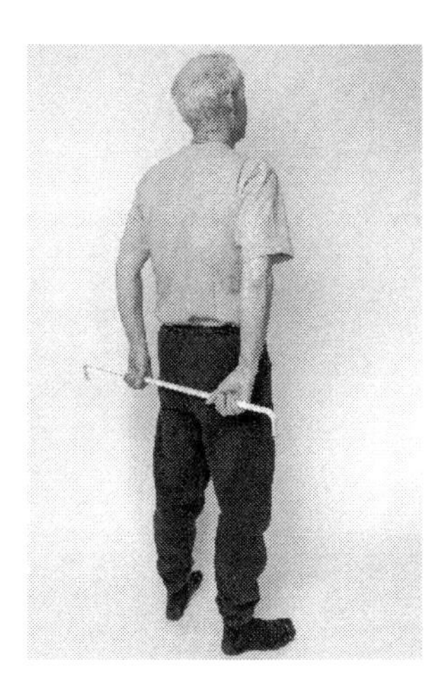

Start

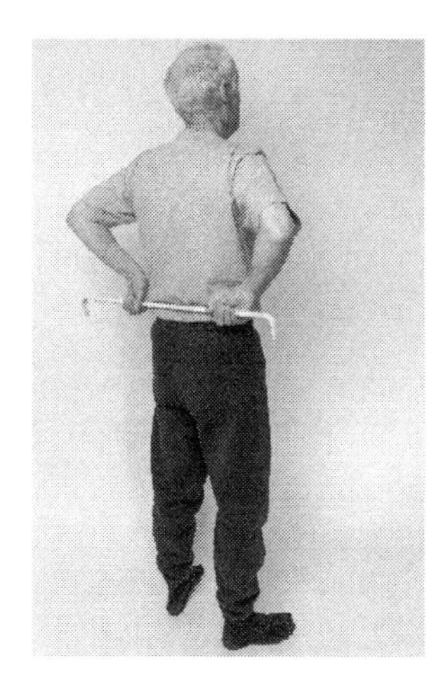

End

Static Lying Flexion

Purpose: Increase ability to reach overhead. One of the six key stretches.

Equipment Needed:

- Blocks for measuring.
- A rod to push/pull with. A bathroom curtain rod about 25 inches long with a 90-degree bend at the end works well for this as described in Appendix 4.

Directions

- Arrange the blocks in a stack on the floor at the desired height.
- (If this is the first time you've done this, then you'll need to determine what the optimal height is. To do that, adjust the height and position of the stack so that after about ten seconds the back of your weak hand comes to rest about one inch above the stack from the pull of gravity alone.)
- Lie down on the floor with the stack about a foot above your head.
- Slowly lift your weak arm over your head and down towards the stack. You can use the rod to help you with this if needed.
- Using the rod, push your hand down the rest of the way so that the back of your hand rests flat on the stack.
- Hold the stretch for 30 seconds as long as there's not too much pain.
- Bring your weak arm back to your body. To make it easier, grasp the rod with your weak hand and let you well arm pull it back.
- Record the height of the stretch in your log.
- After two to five days you can try to increase the stretch by 1/4 inch, but only if you can hold the stretch for the entire 30 seconds without too much pain.
- Note: Take extra care to be consistent when performing this exercise. Try locking your elbow as you do it. As you bring your arm down onto the blocks, just graze your ear with your forearm each time.

See the next page for illustrations.

Static Lying Flexion, Illustrations

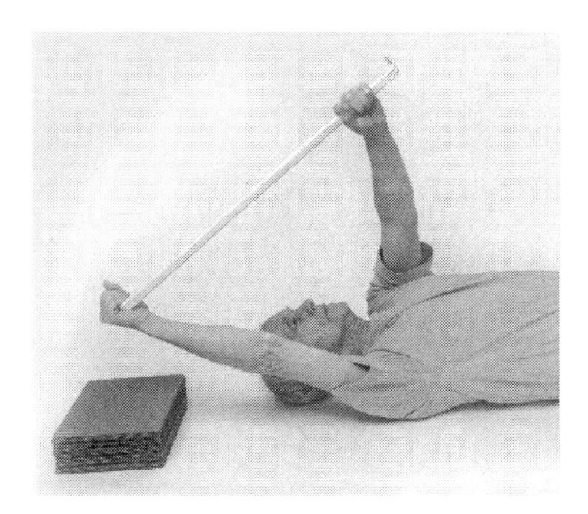

1-Lower arm down towards blocks

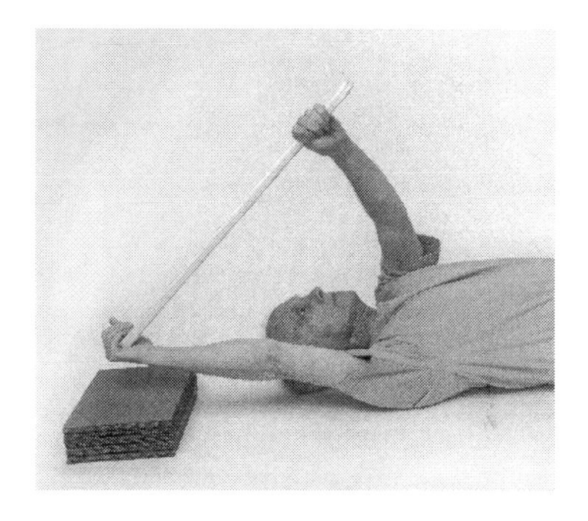

2-Arm 1" above blocks

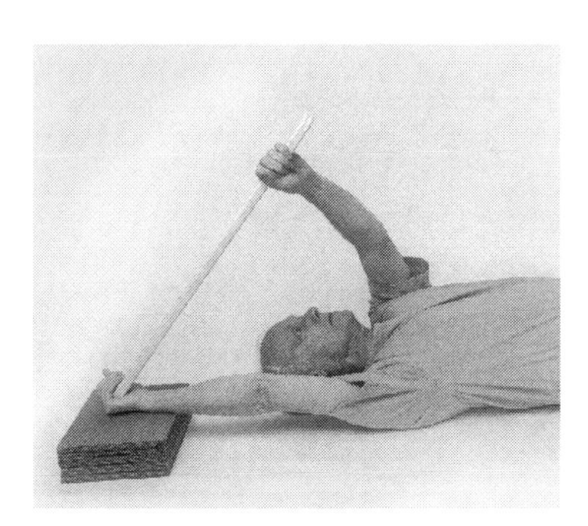

3-Push arm down to blocks and hold

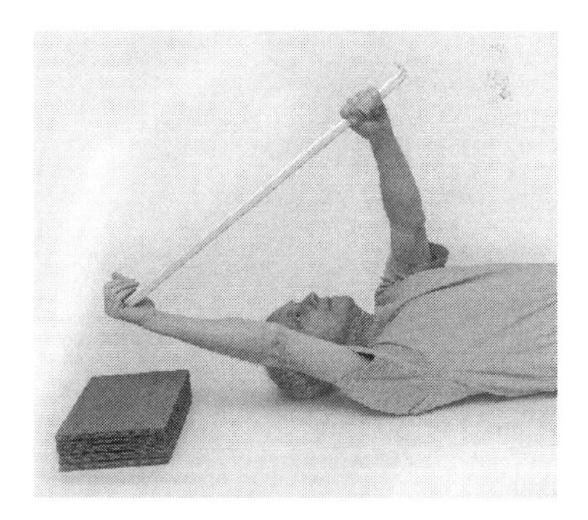

4-Pull arm back

Horizontal External Rotation at Side

Purpose: One of the six key stretches, it will help you with movements used in tennis and table tennis, and also to get you ready for the next exercise.

Equipment Needed:

The same as in the Static Lying Flexion exercise.

Directions

- Arrange blocks on the floor the same height as the last time you did the exercise. If it's been at least two days since the stack height was decreased, you can try lowering it by 1/4 inch as long as it isn't too painful.
- Lie down on the floor with your weak arm pressed lightly against your side and the blocks about ten inches from your elbow. Your forearm should be pointed upwards.
- Rotate your arm down towards the stack of blocks.
- With the rod in your well hand, push your weak hand down onto the stack so that the back of your hand rests flat on the stack. Hold for 30 seconds.
- When you're finished, record the height of the blocks on your log sheet.

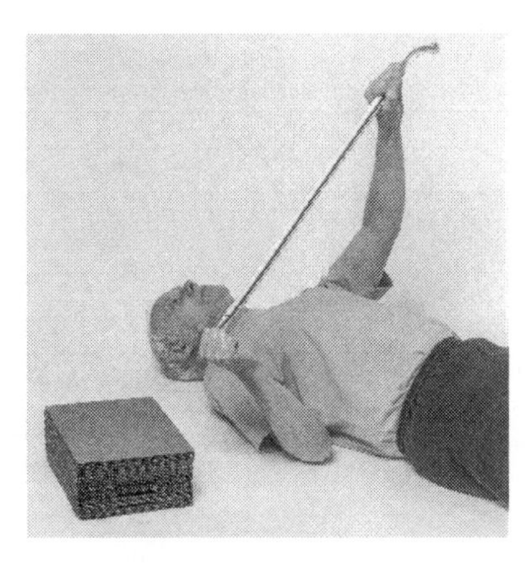

1-Starting position

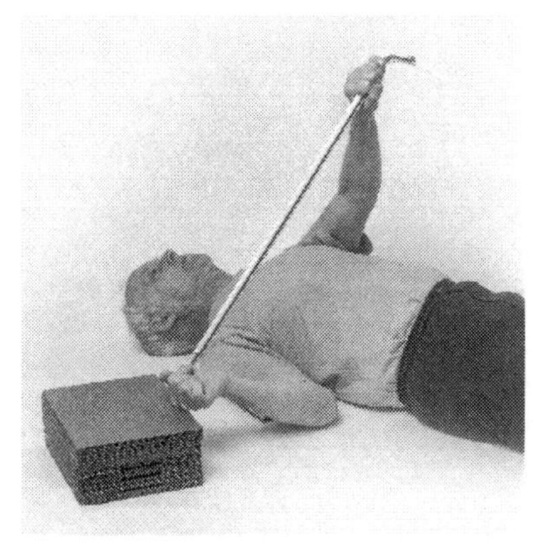

2-Push weak arm down onto blocks

Horizontal External Rotation

Purpose: One of the six key stretches, useful for lifting your arm up and back as in throwing a ball. This exercise could be painful so don't push it too hard.

Equipment Needed:

- Same as for Static Lying Flexion.

Directions

- Arrange blocks on the floor the same height as the last time you did the exercise. If it's been at least two days since the stack height was decreased, you can try lowering it by 1/4 inch as long as it doesn't cause too much pain.
- Lie down on the floor with your shoulder about ten inches to the side and down from the stack. Extend your weak arm out on the floor at a 90 degree angle from your body. Raise your forearm straight up from the floor.
- Push your arm straight down towards the stack. Don't bend your wrist. Your hand should come to rest up to an inch above the stack from gravity alone. Use the rod and your well arm to push it down the rest of the way. Hold the stretch for 30 seconds.
- When you're finished, record the height of the stack on your log sheet.

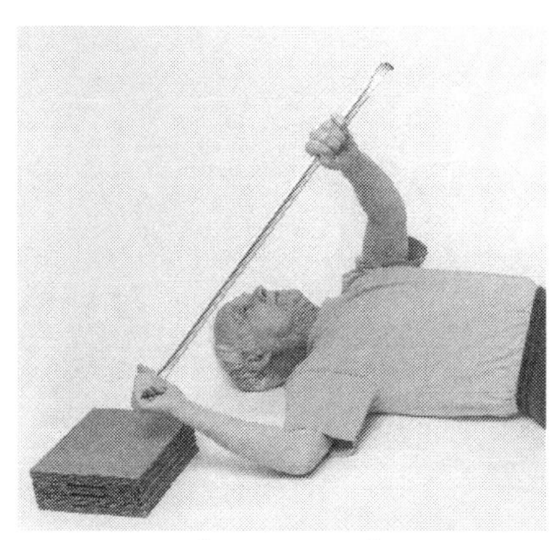

1-Pushing arm down

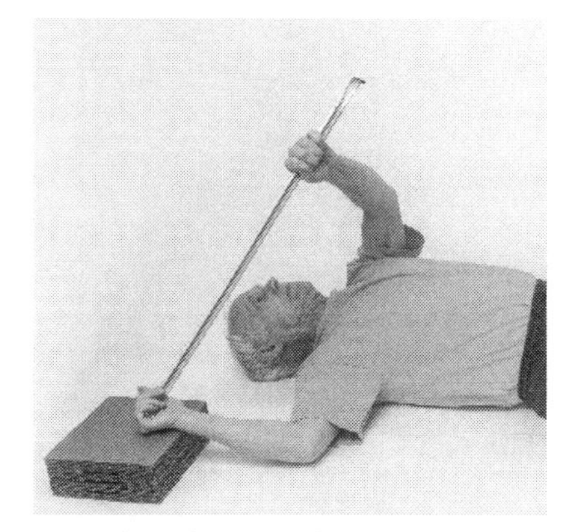

2-End with hand flat on blocks

Horizontal Internal Rotation

Purpose: One of the six key stretches. Works the movement needed to push down on something, such as closing a suitcase that's stuffed full.

Equipment Needed:

- Same as for Lying Flexion.

Directions

- Arrange blocks on the floor the same height as the last time you did the exercise. If it's been two days or more since the stack height was decreased, you can consider lowering it by 1/4 inch.
- Lie down on the floor with your shoulder about ten inches to the side and up from the stack. Stick your weak arm out on the floor at a 90 degree angle from your body with your forearm pointed upwards.
- Lower your weak arm forward straight down towards the stack with the palm of your hand leading. Keep your wrist straight. Your palm should come to rest up to an inch above the stack. Use the rod and your well arm to push it down the rest of the way.
- When you're finished, record the amount of stretch on your log sheet.

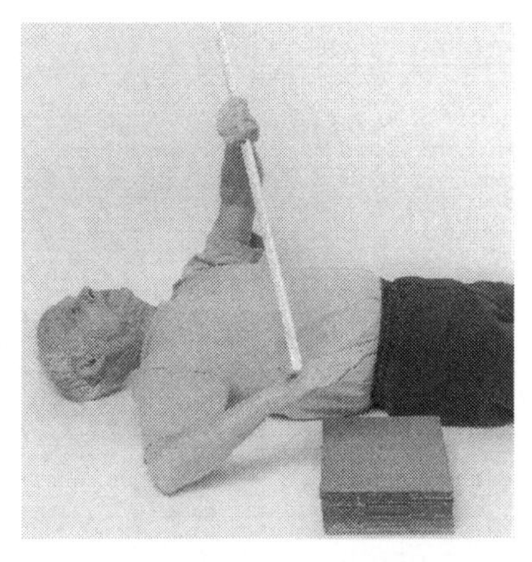

1-Push arm down towards blocks

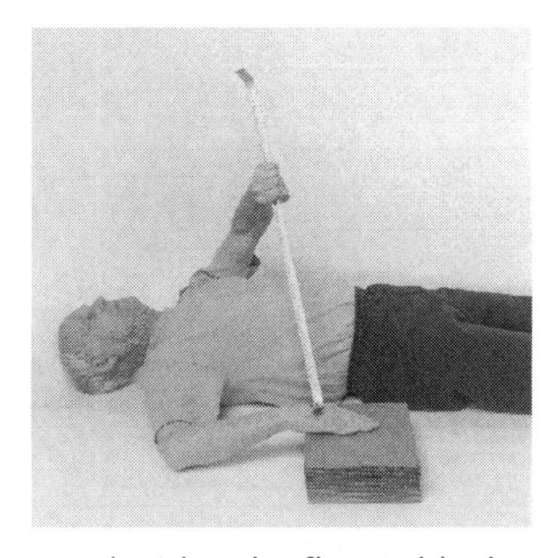

2-End with palm flat on blocks

Pulley Stretch (Passive Flexion)

Purpose: Increase ability to reach overhead. This is a passive stretch where the well arm is used to give the weak arm a good stretch.

Equipment Needed:

- A pulley made for this purpose and a place to mount the pulley, such as over a door, a beam in your house or garage, a gazebo, a pergola, a tree limb, etc.
- Tape to mark the extent of your current stretch. Painter's tape works well.

Directions

- Depending on where you've mounted the pulley and your preferences, you can sit or stand while doing this stretch. The key is to sit or stand in the same relation to the pulley each time so that your stretch is consistent.
- Grasp the handles of the pulley with each hand. Pull down with the well hand which will pull the weak arm up. Stop at the point where you previously marked your high point. (The high point can be marked by wrapping a little piece of tape around the rope adjacent to the handle in your weak hand.)
- Hold the stretch for 30 seconds.
- When you can easily reach the mark, move it up higher by 1/4 inch.

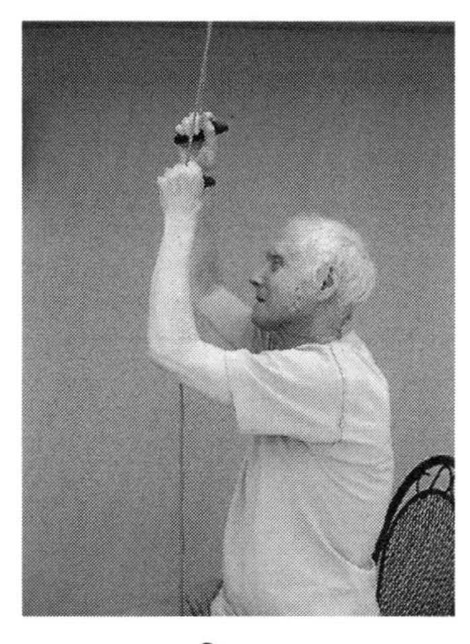

Start

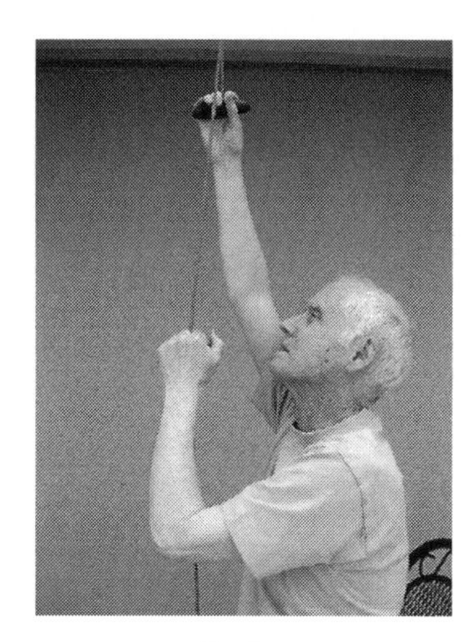

End

Abduction (Angels)

Purpose: One of the key stretches. Improves ability to raise arm straight out from side as in basketball to block your opponent's shot.

Equipment Needed:
- Therapy strap. See Appendix 4 for further information.

Directions
- Take the therapy strap and sit down on the floor.
- Put your foot on your weak side through the loop in the strap.
- Grasp the strap at the mark where you left off in your previous stretch. If it's been at least two days since you last increased the stretch, consider moving your grip half an inch to an inch higher on the strap.
- Lie down on your back and extent your leg on your weak side straight down from your waist.
- Extend your weak arm straight out from your side.
- Keeping your arm on the floor, move your arm up towards your head until the strap becomes taught.
- Hold the stretch in that position for 30 seconds.
- Record the stretch on your log sheet.

See the next page for illustrations.

Abduction (Angels), Illustrations

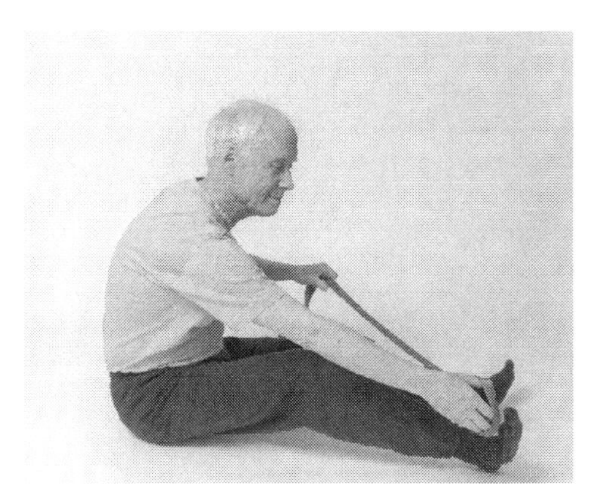

1-Put foot through loop

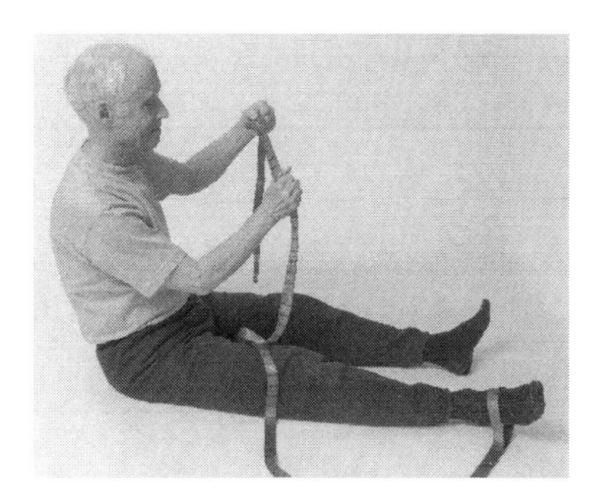

2-Grasp the strap at
the desired mark

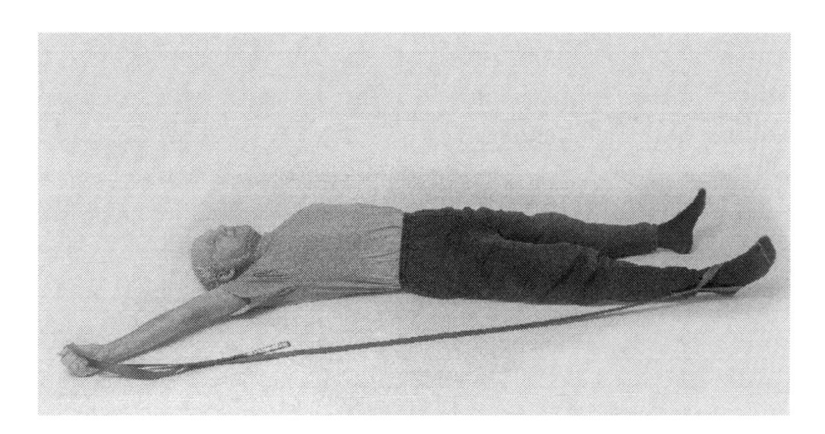

3-Move your arm upwards until
the strap becomes taut

Internal Rotation behind the Back

Purpose: Improves ability to do motions behind the back such as scratching or tucking in your shirt. One of the six key exercises. Note: this exercise may be very painful at first. If so, then do the dynamic exercises Standing Extension with Rod and Standing Internal Rotation with Rod until you can do this one more easily.

Equipment Needed: Therapy strap. See Appendix 4 for further information.

Directions

- Stand in front of a mirror. Drop the loop of the strap over your well shoulder so that the inch markings show in the mirror.
- Lower the strap down your back to where you can put your weak hand through the loop and adjust the loop at your wrist.
- Make a fist with your weak hand and try and place your knuckles somewhere along your spine.
- Now, pull and lift your arm up at least as far as your last stretch while keeping your knuckles at your spine.
- Hold the stretch for 30 seconds.
- To measure the distance of your stretch, you can lean forward and read the measurement right at the ridge line of your shoulder. Because of the viewing angle when looking in a mirror, it's easier to record your measurements in inches rather than 1/4 inches.
- Alternatively, if you have someone else around who can help, they can read the measurement for you. If you have a helper, they may be able to read the number to an accuracy of half an inch. They can also help you slip your hand through the loop. This is where the buddy system can really be useful.
- This can be a painful exercise, so wait to increase the stretch until you can do so comfortably.
- The measurements of this stretch can vary by an inch or so just by wearing different weights of clothing. For best results, try and wear similar clothing every time you do this stretch. See the next page for illustrations.

Internal Rotation behind the Back, Illustrations

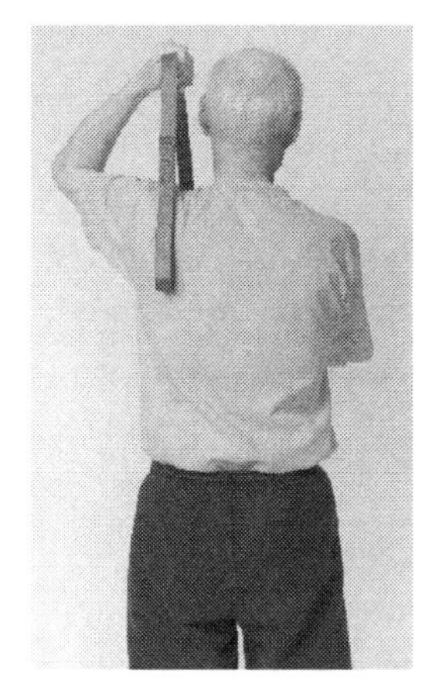

1-Drop loop end of strap over well shoulder

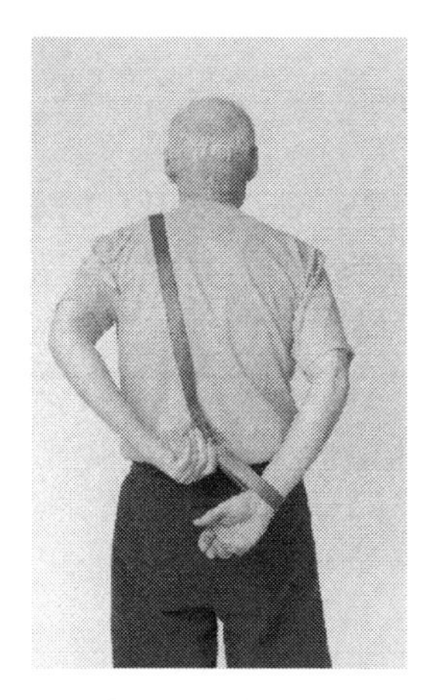

2-Slip weak hand through loop

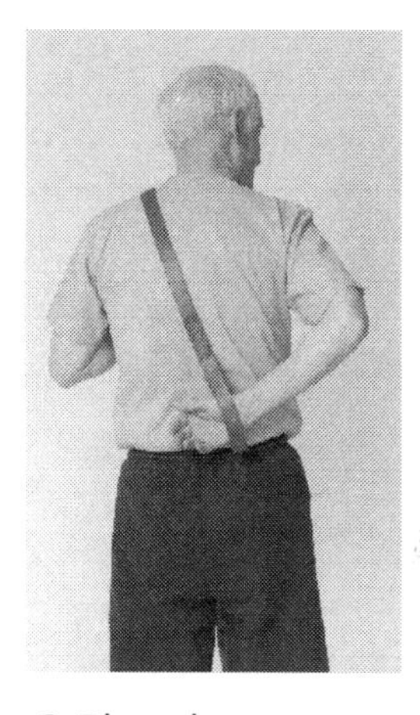

3-Place loop at wrist and knuckles at spine

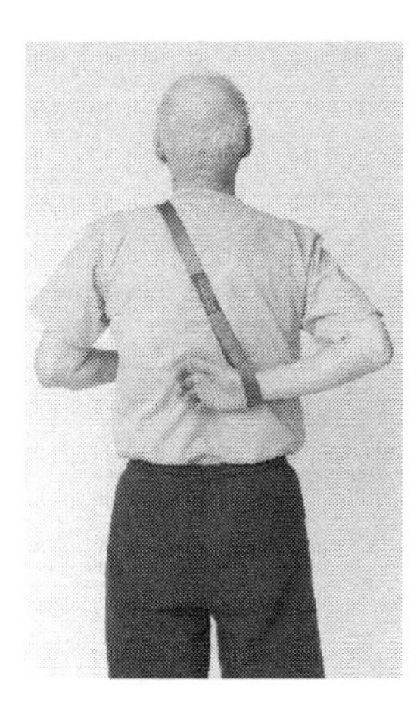

4-Pull and lift arm up to desired height

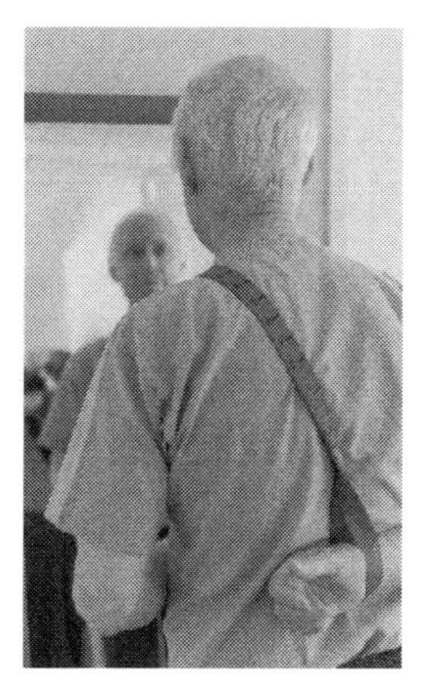

5-Look in mirror and read the inch scale at your shoulder ridge

Wall Reach (Standing Flexion)

Purpose: A convenient flexion exercise that can be done passively or actively.

Equipment Needed: A strip of painter's tape, a ruler, and a marking pen. Put a vertical strip of painter's tape on a wall or door jamb as high up as your well arm can reach and extending down beyond where your weak arm can reach. Reaching up as high as you can with your well arm, make a mark with your pen. With your ruler, draw a vertical line from that point down to where your weak arm can reach. With the bottom of the line as zero, make a major mark every inch up the tape, and a minor mark every 1/4 inch. Number the inch marks.

Directions

- Reach the fingertips of your weak arm up to your target mark. Hold the stretch for 30 seconds.
- This exercise can also be done more passively in a couple of ways: one is simply to grasp your weak arm with your well hand and assist your weak arm to slide up the wall. Another variation is to use the fingers of your weak hand to "walk" up the wall, taking your weak arm with it.
- Consider logging your progress on this exercise and try to extend your reach periodically per the guidelines in chapter 8.

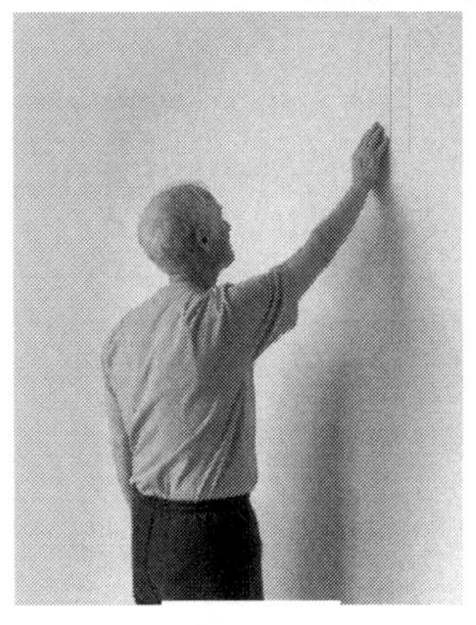

Start

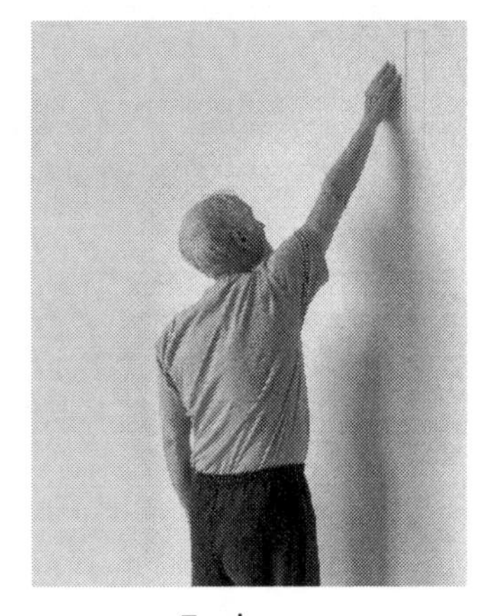

End

Part Three:

Strengthening Exercises

10—Build Strength Effectively

We lose range of motion (ROM) in our shoulders because of stiffness, pain, and muscle weakness. The four muscles associated with the rotator cuff are relatively small so that if they become weak they may be unable to move the shoulder through its full range of motion. (The *rotator cuff* is described in Appendix 1.) Therefore, it's good to start some mild strengthening exercises as soon as we can as long as it doesn't cause pain. If pain is felt in any particular exercise, then skip it and do one that can be done without pain. ***If all of the exercises are painful, then continue with mild stretching exercises until the strength training can be done without pain.*** When in doubt, consult with your practitioner about this.

When we write of "strength training exercises" we mean exercises done against a resistance of some sort, such as elastic bands, weights, or pressing against a fixed object. There are two general ways of classifying strength training exercises:

Isotonic exercise involves contracting our muscles so that they become shorter and then longer again as we do the exercise. We can tell an exercise is isotonic when our limbs move. An example of this would be rowing.

Isometric exercise involves contracting a muscle, but the limb doesn't move during the contraction so that the joint angle and muscle length remain the same. An example of this would be an arm-wrestling contest between two perfectly matched contestants where neither of their arms move much.

The advantage to isotonic exercises is that our progress can be easily and accurately tracked, especially with weights. We know how many pounds we are lifting and can express it as a number. The disadvantage to them is that they do require special equipment which costs money, requires storage space, and can be inconvenient when we are traveling.

Isometric exercises have at least three advantages. Since the shoulder doesn't move when we are doing them, they may be less likely to cause injury. Since they don't require special equipment, they are easier to do when traveling. Finally, if you're shoulder injury is relatively new, especially if it's a rotator cuff tear, you may be able to do mild isometric exercises without pain so you could start out with those. However, there are a couple of disadvantages. With isometrics, usually all we can go by is the feel, which doesn't lend itself to consistency and constant progress. Another negative is that if we overexert ourselves, they may raise our blood pressure more than the isotonic exercises do, which can be dangerous.

In general, we prefer the isotonic exercises, and they are what we present in this book. However, if you are traveling and don't have access to exercise equipment, then some isometric exercises would help to keep you in shape until you get back home. For example, internal and external rotation exercises can easily be done by exerting pressure against a door jamb. When doing these exercises, we recommend that you do up to 30 repetitions and exert pressure for about three seconds. Do this once a day, three times per week.

There are a multitude of exercises that can be done in a variety of positions including standing, sitting, lying on your back or your stomach. We offer here a starter set that will condition all four of your rotator cuff muscles as well as various other muscles that are used in shoulder motion. There are plenty of other exercises that you can find for free on the internet, such as from the American Association of Orthopedic Surgeons (see Resources). At some point you may want to do some others for variety. However, if the exercises look especially difficult or awkward, be sure to consult with your practitioner about their suitability and how to execute them with the correct form.

When doing resistance exercises, you can go at your own pace, but keep the movements smooth and steady so that you don't hurt your shoulder. Avoid any jerky movements. For example, if using an elastic band, don't relax and let the band snap your arm back to the starting position.

Additional concepts used in strength training are *sets* and *repetitions* (reps). Repetitions are a count of how many times in a row we do a particular exercise without stopping. Sets are groups of repetitions. For example, if we do ten repetitions of an exercise, rest for 30 seconds, then do another group of ten repetitions, we have done two sets of ten repetitions. In this book we recommend doing just one set for each given exercise. This should be enough for rehabilitation purposes to gain enough strength to move your arm through its full range of motion.

In doing resistance training, we also have to decide whether our goal is to build *strength, endurance*, or a balance between the two. To build a lot of strength requires a high-intensity workout which can lead to reinjury. Therefore, in this book, we lean towards building endurance more than strength which should enable most people to get back to their normal life. For the serious athletes and body builders, once they have successfully rehabilitated their shoulders, they can follow up with their coaches to keep progressing towards their goals.

In order to build endurance, we use less resistance, but we do a higher number of reps. In our program, we recommend starting out an exercise with enough resistance that we can do the movement ten times before getting exhausted and/or feeling pain. We then gradually build up the number of reps until we can do 20. At that point we increase the resistance—say by one pound—drop the reps back down to ten, and repeat the process. Following is a sample of what we mean:

Week	Weight Lbs.	Sets	Reps
1	2	1	10
2	2	1	13
3	2	1	16
4	2	1	20
5	3	1	10
6	3	1	13
Etc.			

A general guideline for rehabilitation purposes is to work our way up to a resistance equal to four percent of body weight. This may not seem like much, but remember that the rotator cuff muscles are relatively small, so we really want to avoid overstressing them. The exercises are not meant to increase muscle mass, but to get us back to full range of motion and nothing more. Also, remember that this is just a general guideline. With some easier exercises, such as internal rotation, you might be able to use greater resistance, but with harder exercises, such as seated horizontal external rotation, you should probably use less. *When in doubt, we recommend that you confirm with your practitioner what a suitable goal would be for a given exercise given your age, body build, the nature of your injury, and how far along you are in the healing process.*

In general, we prefer to use fixed weights to do strength training unless a particular exercise is awkward that way, in which case we switch to resistance bands. (See discussions of this equipment in Appendix 4 under "Resistance Bands" and "Weights.") In order to keep our bodies balanced, we also like to do the exercises with *both* arms. In that case, it's convenient to have two dumbbells available, one for each hand.

Start with the resistance level that you can handle without pain and without soreness afterwards. One rule of thumb is called the ***2-hour rule,*** which states that if there is any soreness two hours after doing an exercise, then you have overdone it.

Strengthening Routine

Below is a list of the strengthening exercises presented in this book. Remember to record your progress with each exercise as you do it. A sample strength training log form is included in Appendix 6; feel free to copy it or devise your own form. Each exercise description lists the muscles worked. Appendix 1 describes where the four rotator cuff shoulder muscles are located, but other muscles listed in the exercises are not described in this book. Strength training exercises should be done two or three times per week, depending upon your condition and how well your body responds to the exercises. Don't do strength training two days in a row; there should be a day or two of rest between strength training sessions. Note that the exercises don't have to be done in the order below; if you prefer doing them in a different order, that's okay.

1. Warm Up

Do the same pendulum exercises that you did to warm up for stretching.

2. Strengthening Exercises

Internal rotation with Resistance Band
Standing low row
Standing diagonal dumbbell raise
Scaption
External rotation at side
Side lying Abduction
Seated horizontal external rotation

3. Cool Down

Apply Ice for up to 15 minutes.

11—Strength Training Exercises

Internal Rotation with Resistance Band

Muscles worked: Subscapularis and pectoralis
Equipment Needed: One resistance tube or band. (For convenience, we'll just refer to bands in the instructions.) Small folded towel (optional).

Directions

- Anchor the band to a door or other fixed object.
- Stand in a relaxed position with the shoulder that you are working pointed towards the band's anchor.
- Grasp the band keeping your elbow down at your side, and forearm extended horizontally out in front of you and a bit to the side.
- For less stress and greater comfort in doing the exercise, try putting a folded towel between the arm and body of the shoulder you are working.
- Now, slowly bend your forearm in towards your stomach and pause. Then, slowly reverse the movement back to the starting position. Stay in control at all times and don't let the band snap your arm back.

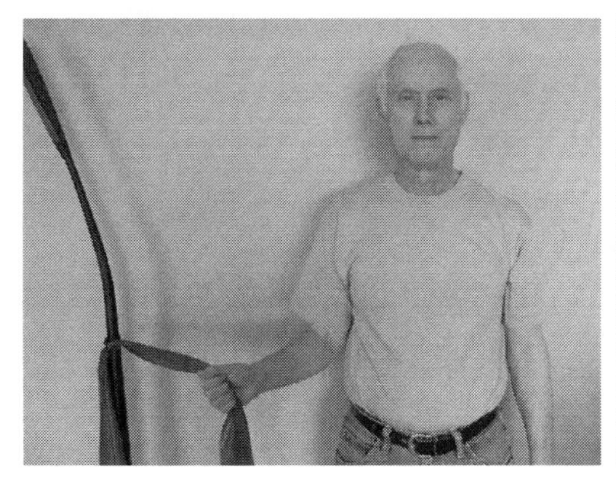

Start

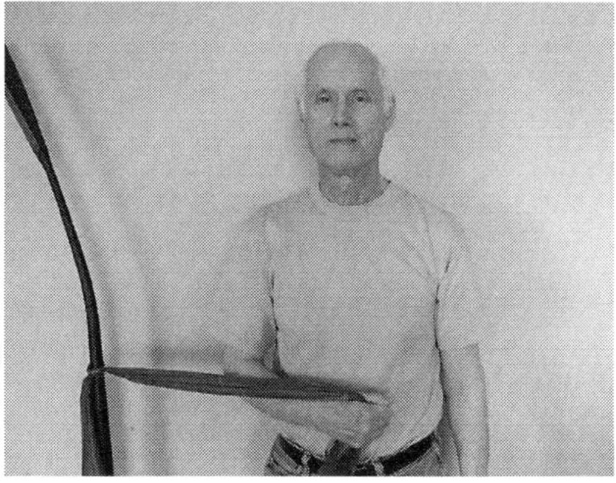

End

Standing Low Row

Muscles worked: Middle and lower trapezius, deltoids, rhomboids
Equipment Needed: Resistance tubes or bands. Anchor resistance bands to door or other solid object at about waist level.

Directions

- Stand with feet shoulder width apart, knees slightly bent. Grasp bands with both hands, arms extended in front with elbows slightly bent.
- Pull bands back towards your body, stopping when elbows reach your sides. It's also good to squeeze your shoulder blades together a bit as you pull back to keep your rotator cuff capsule from constricting.

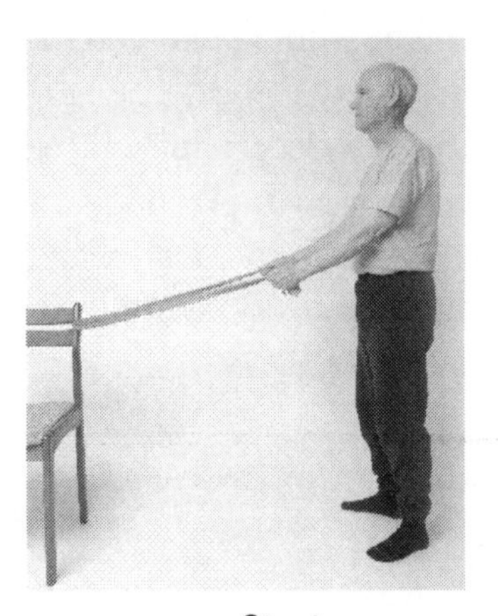

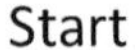

Start

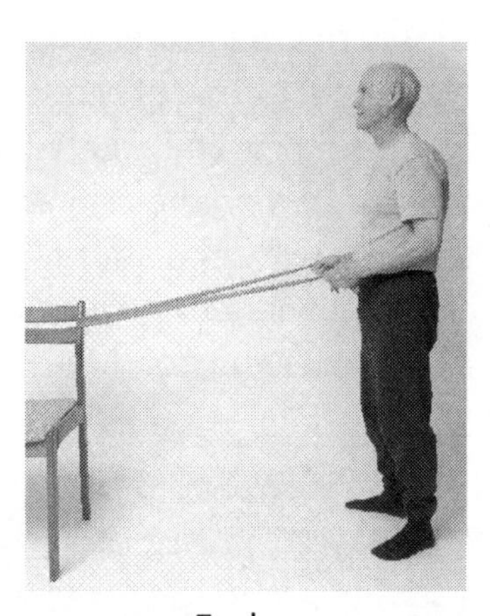

End

Variations:
High Row: Start with your elbows raised up almost to shoulder height and keep them at that height as you pull your arms back.
Sitting Row: Anchor bands to solid object near floor or around your own outstretched foot. Sit down and pull back with rowing motion.
Lat Pull Down: Anchor bands high up such as at the top of a door. Be seated and pull bands down to your chest with your elbows out from your sides.

Standing Diagonal Dumbbell Raise

Muscles worked: All four rotator cuff muscles.

Equipment Needed: One dumbbell. Make sure the weight is moderate.

Directions

- Stand comfortably in a stable position.
- Starting position: Grasp the dumbbell and move your arm diagonally and low across your body towards the opposite thigh.
- Slowly lift the weight diagonally upwards and out in front of you continuing the movement upwards to a 45 degree angle out as far to your side as you can go without pain.
- Do ten to 20 reps, switch hands, and do the other arm.

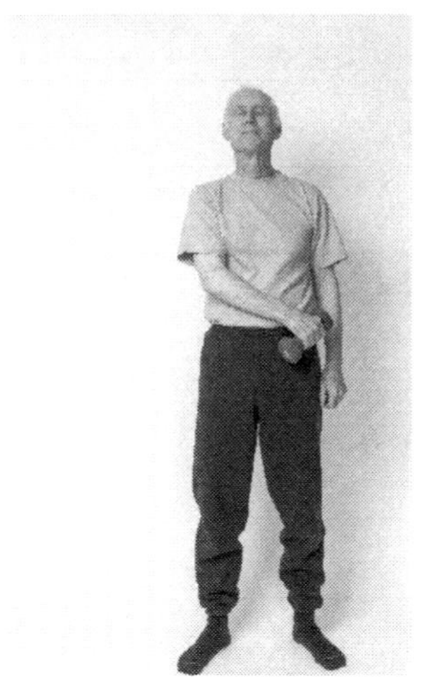

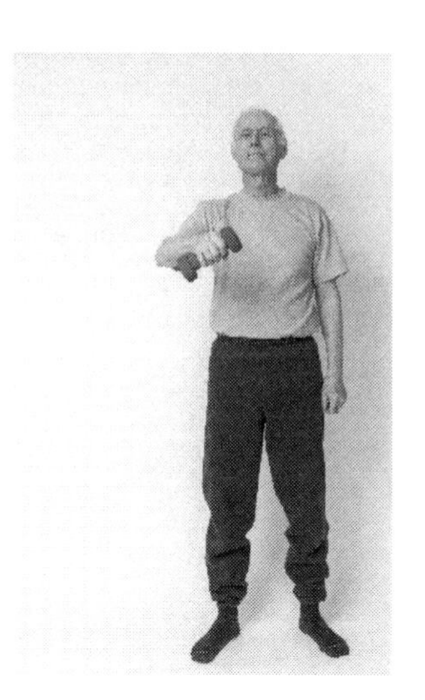

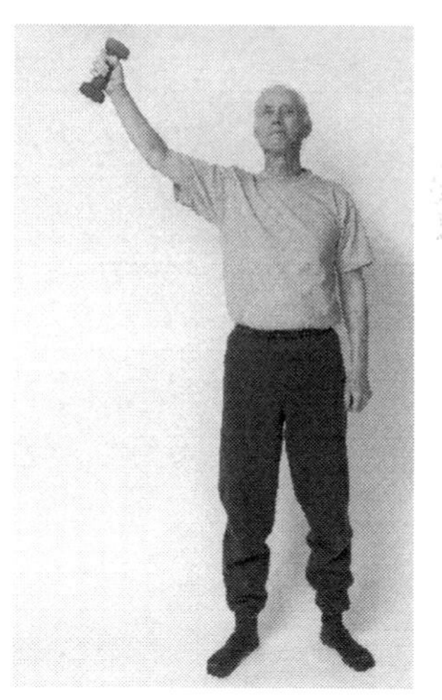

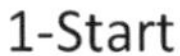

1-Start 2-Half Way 3-End

Scaption

Muscles worked: Supraspinatus, a slow-to-heal, commonly-affected rotator cuff muscle. This is a strenuous exercise, so be sure to go slowly with it. It's best to start out just lifting your arms with no weights and work up from there. Discontinue the exercise if pain or weakness last for more than two hours.

Equipment Needed: One dumbbell for each hand with weight that is not too heavy.

Directions

- Stand in a relaxed position with feet shoulder width apart for good balance.
- Hold the dumbbells in a comfortable position with the palms of your hands pointed towards each other.
- Hold your arms low and away from your body at approximately a 30 to 45 degree angle.
- Now, slowly lift your arms up to shoulder height counting 1, 2, 3, 4; slight pause, and down 1, 2, 3, 4 and relax.

See illustrations on next page.

Scaption, Illustrations

Side Views

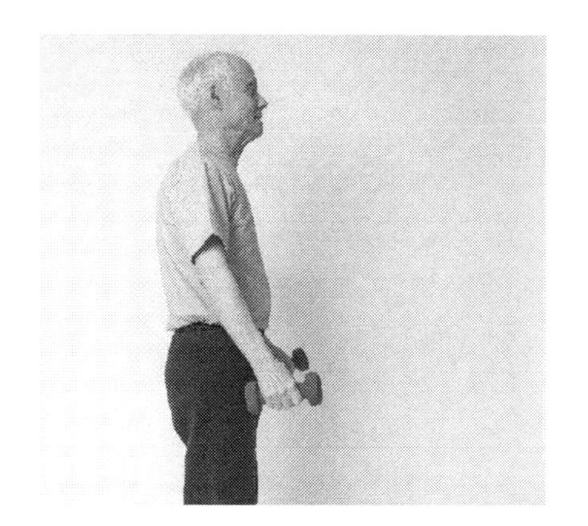

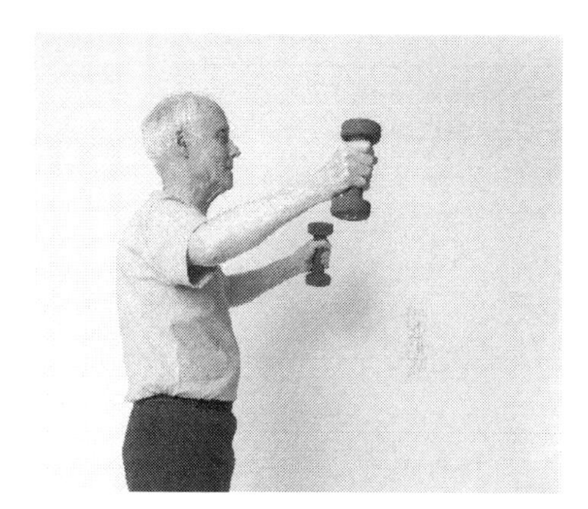

Front Views

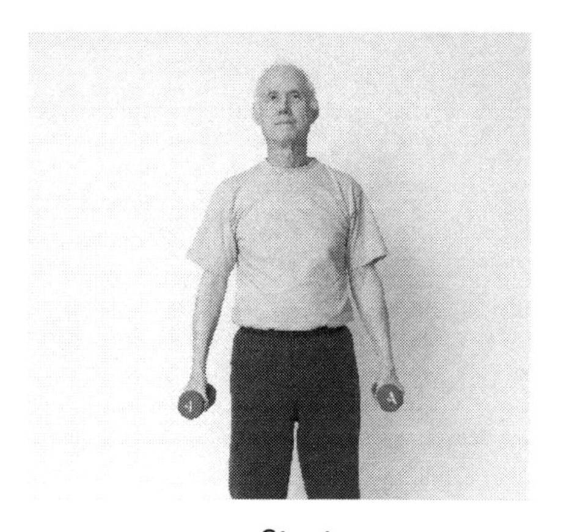

Start

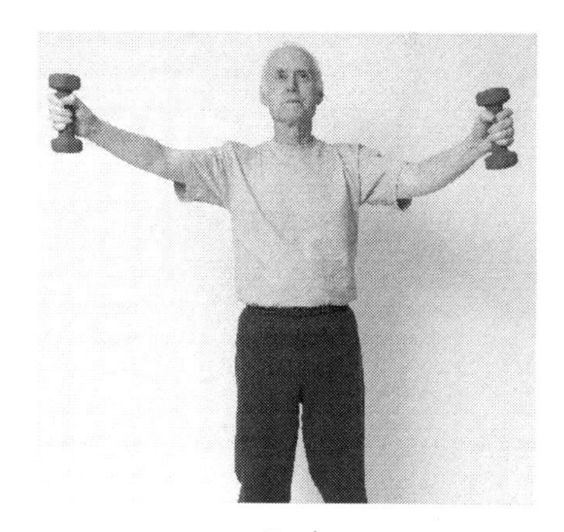

End

External Rotation at Side

Muscles worked: Infraspinatus and teres minor.

Equipment Needed: One dumbbell and folded towel.

Directions

- Lie down on your side.
- Hold your arm at your side and the towel between your upper arm and your side. Your forearm should be at a 90 degree angle and extending down and away from your body.
- Slowly lift the weight straight up as far as you can, then slowly straight down. Avoid overdoing it at the top of the lift where the stress is greatest.
- Note: This exercise can also be done standing up using bands. For example, if you're exercising your well arm, you might want to avoid lying on your weak arm. The next page shows how to do the exercise using bands.

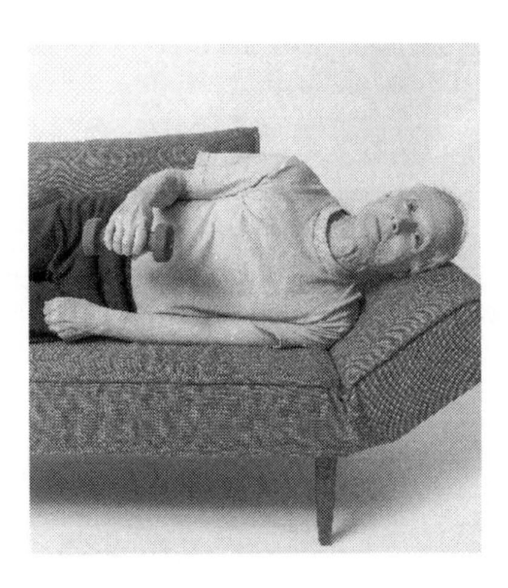

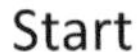

Start

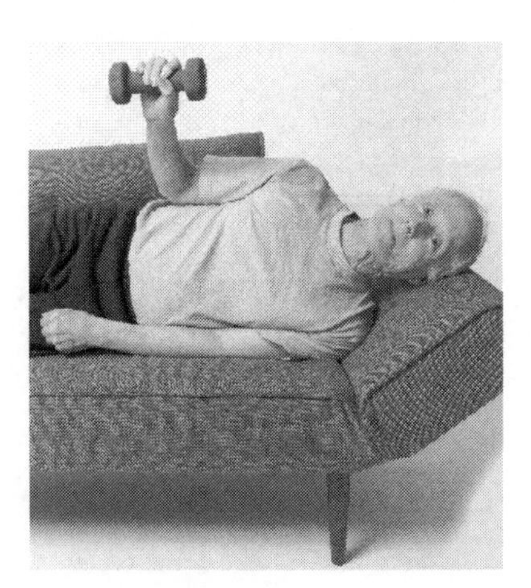

End

External Rotation with Resistance Band

Muscles worked: Infraspinatus and teres minor.

Equipment Needed: One resistance tube or band. Optional folded towel.

Directions

- Anchor the band to a door or other fixed object.
- Stand in a relaxed position with the shoulder that you are working pointed away from the band's anchor.
- Grasp the band keeping your elbow down at your side, and forearm extended horizontally towards your tummy.
- For less stress and greater comfort in doing the exercise, try putting a folded towel between the arm and body of the shoulder you are working.
- Now, slowly rotate your forearm away from your body and pause. Then, slowly reverse the movement back to the starting position. Stay in control at all times and don't let the band snap your arm back.

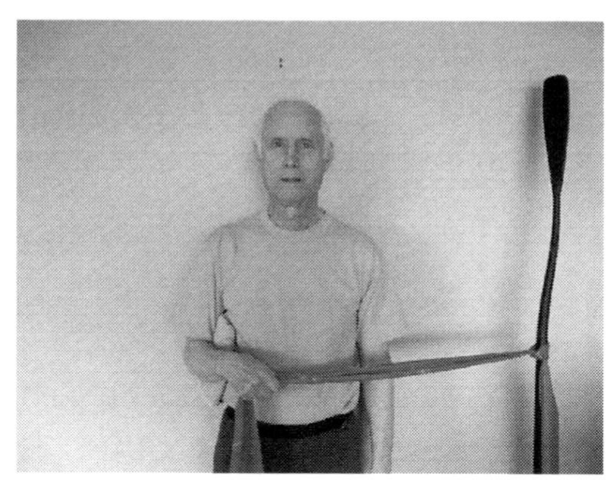

Start

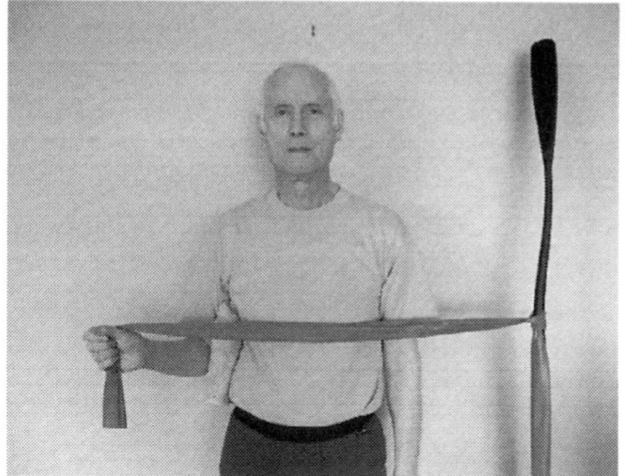

End

Side Lying Abduction

Muscles worked: Supraspinatus and serratus anterior.

Equipment Needed: One dumbbell.

Directions

- Lie down on your well side.
- Start with your weak arm at your side, holding the dumbbell.
- Slowly lift the weight straight up from your side until your arm makes about a 45 degree angle with your body. Lower your arm slowly to your side.
- Do between ten and 20 reps.
- If doing both arms, switch sides and repeat.
- If it hurts to lie on your weak side, try doing it standing instead.

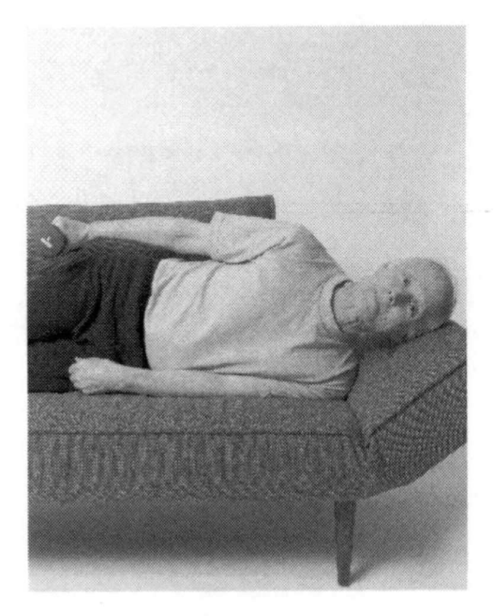

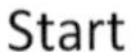
Start

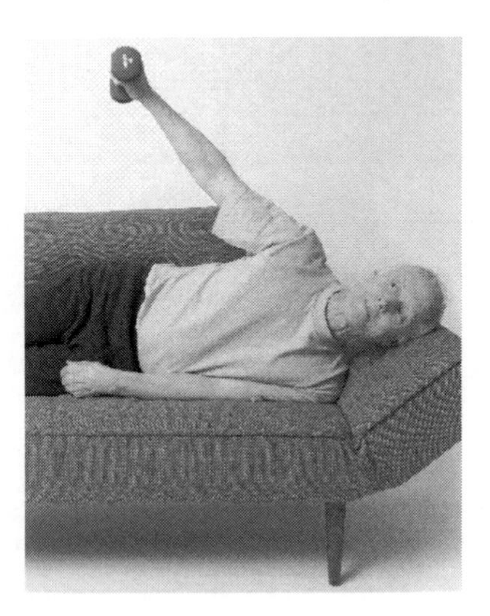
End

Seated Horizontal External Rotation

Muscles worked: Infraspinatus, teres minor, and posterior deltoid.
Equipment Needed: One dumbbell.

Directions

- Sit comfortably beside a sofa or other item where you are able to extend your arm out horizontally from your side and rest your elbow it.
- Bend your elbow to make a 90 degree angle with your forearm pointed straight out in front of you with the palm pointed down and rest your elbow on the sofa.
- Slowly lift the weight straight up towards the ceiling as high as you can without undue strain.
- Slowly lower again and repeat ten to 20 times. Make sure your elbow stays in line with your shoulder.
- Remember that it's preferable to work both arms.
- We recommend that you not try and do this exercise without a support as that would put a lot of strain on your shoulder.

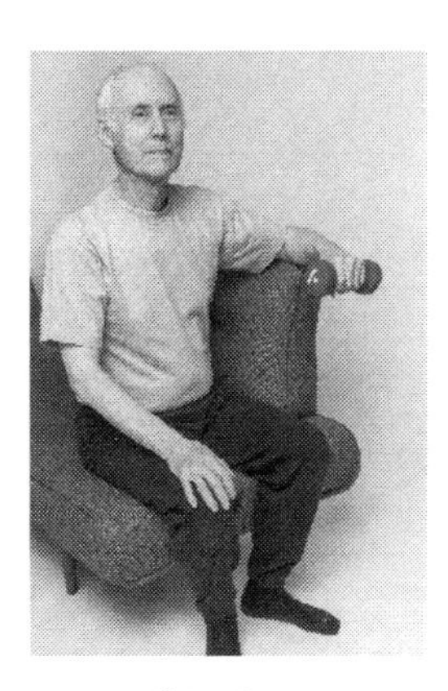

Start

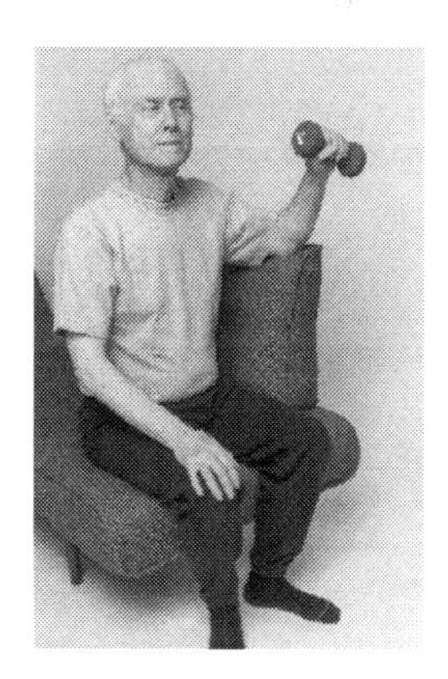

End

Part Four:

Maintenance

12—Maintenance

Once our shoulder is healed, it's definitely worth some time and effort to keep the problem from coming back. If we have a recurrence, not only do we have to spend the time and energy required to recover, but the second time around we may not recover as fully, either. As we mentioned in chapter 1, once we've had a shoulder injury, we may be 27% more likely to have a recurrence. Therefore, extra effort is advised to avoid that scenario. Following is a list of steps you can take to minimize the chances of reinjury.

1. Stay in the *green* zone. In discussing ROM, some experts divide the movements that we move our arms through up into *green*, *yellow* and *red* zones. In the green zone, we are generally safe from injuring our shoulder other than through overuse. In the yellow zone, we don't have as much margin for error; injury is possible, and we need to be careful. In the red zone injury is even more likely, especially if our arm is moved into this position through an abrupt and intense force. The best bet is to strive to always stay in the green zone in our daily life. About the only excuse for venturing into the red zone would be in an emergency situation, such as rescuing someone from a dangerous situation. We enter the yellow zone for a specific purpose, such as when we are trying to increase our ROM through stretching exercises, but as we have emphasized, this is done in a very cautious way so that we don't overextend ourselves.

So where are these zones? They are specific to each individual based upon their age, any history of previous injuries, and the general flexibility that they were born with. However, there are some general rules of thumb that we can use as a starting point and then fine tune from there to determine our individual zones. The zones can be divided up into three categories are follows:

Flexion zone. This is for movements of the arm straight out in front of us and up towards the sky as when children are raising their hands in school. The rule of thumb is that as the arm moves from hanging down at our side to straight out in front of us as if pointing at something, then that is the green zone. As we move the arm from a horizontal position to straight up towards the sky, then that 90 degree movement is all in the yellow zone. Any continuation of the movement from straight up and then back behind our head is in the red zone. To determine the boundary between your particular green and yellow zone, start with your hands at your sides with the palms of your hands towards your thighs. Raise your hands slowly up in front of you towards the ceiling, keeping your palms facing. When you start to feel pain or stiffness, you are entering the yellow zone. Note that the zones may be different for each arm.

Abduction zone. If you hold your arms horizontally straight out in front of you with your palms facing and then move your arms away from each other straight back keeping them in the horizontal plane, then that movement is called *abduction*. If you are standing with your back against a wall, then the rule of thumb is that your arms would be in the green zone all the way back to where your arms are touching the wall. Up to another 20 degrees beyond that would be in the yellow zone, and beyond that would be the red zone. To determine your own individual green zone, do this exercise yourself and note if there is any pain or stiffness as you move your arms back towards the wall. If you encounter resistance before reaching the wall, then you are now in the yellow zone. Ten to 20 degrees beyond that would put you in the red zone—don't go there!

Extension zone. When your arms are hanging down at your sides and you move them straight back behind you, then that movement is called *extension*. It's the reverse of flexion; it's the kind of motion we do when we're bowling. This motion is the most restricted of the three motions, and hence the most dangerous. The rule of thumb for extension is that the average person should be able to move her arms back about 25 degrees, or around eight inches depending on the length of the arms. The yellow zone for this movement is very small, perhaps another 4 inches or ten degrees or so. Beyond that would be the red zone. When we have a shoulder problem this motion may be very restricted and painful and we can't even enter what is typically considered the green zone. Hopefully, your therapy will give you access to the green zone, but please be aware of any discomfort in this motion and don't go beyond your pain threshold.

2. Cut back on, modify, or eliminate activities that can hurt you.

Examples:
Cut back: Reduce the number of chin-ups you do from 20 to ten.
Modify: Do chin-ups using a machine that reduces the amount of weight you're lifting.
Eliminate: Stop doing chin-ups.

3. Practice good posture.
This is discussed in chapter 4.

4. Shopping
At the grocery store, ensure that the bags are only filled half full. Take extra bags to the store if need be. Make an extra trip from the car to the house to avoid carrying too much at one time, or get a cart to carry the groceries in.

5. Lift properly. The same lifting techniques that we use to protect our backs also apply to our shoulders. To lift properly

- Place your feet shoulder-width apart with one foot slightly in front of the other.
- Hold the load close to your body and lift slowly by straightening your hips and knees.
- Don't twist while you lift, and don't lift heavy loads above shoulder height.

How to lift properly may be easiest to understand by seeing a video on it. Try searching for "Safe Lifting." One video we liked was by "PhoenixParks."

6. Carry properly. For personal items that you carry around for long periods of time in a purse or bag, the best solution is to replace the bag with a fanny pack. The second best choice is to use a bag with a strap that is long enough to comfortably sling across your body and over your well shoulder.

7. Vacuuming, mowing the lawn, sweeping, shoveling snow, etc. With these activities, keep your arms close to your sides. Move your whole body and move your arms less and your legs more. If there are any kids around who might like to do these chores for pay, consider hiring them.

8. Avoid leaning. Do you ever lie down on your side with your arm out and bent, propping your head up while you read, watch TV, or play a game? Do you lie or sit propping yourself up with your elbow, forearm, and shoulder? This is hard on any shoulder, especially a hurt one. This practice should be avoided.

9. Sleep properly. We spend many hours lying in bed, so don't overlook the effect that sleep time can have on your shoulder. The most straight-forward way to reduce harm to your shoulder is simply not to lie on the weak shoulder. To take it a step further, when lying on your well side, it often helps to use a second pillow in one of two positions: one way is to hug a second pillow to your chest with your weak arm draped comfortably over the pillow. This should help to decompress the shoulder capsule and make it feel better. A second way is to lay a thin pillow on top of you on your side and place your weak arm on top of that.

If you simply must lie on your weak side from time to time, then there are ways to mitigate the stress on your shoulder. One way is to use folded blankets or a pillow arranged from your arm pit down to your hip so that more of the pressure is on your trunk and less on your shoulder. You could also try a body pillow. Just search for "body pillow" on Google or Amazon.

10. Take a break every 15 minutes. This is to avoid overuse injuries—stressing our muscles, joints, eyes, etc. without allowing them time to recover. If you're sitting, then stand up and stretch. Lie down and do back stretches if you can. It's also an opportunity to put your back against a wall and check your posture.

Likewise, if you're standing for a long time such as when cooking, take a time-out for a minute and lie down and stretch the back.

11. Use heat before exercising. There's nothing like the moist heat of a brief shower to loosen up and relax the muscles as a way of preventing injuries. This may seem backwards as the usual practice is to shower to wash off the sweat *after* exercising, but swimmers do it all the time. Granted, the main reason for their showers is to keep the water in the pool clean, but it's also a great way to loosen up the muscles.

12. Use ice after exercising. This is optional, but if it makes your shoulder feel better after a workout, then it's probably good for it.

13. Continue with shoulder strength training. As we noted in chapter 2, we may start to lose muscle tone after 72 hours of inactivity. Therefore, it's best to continue with these exercises once or twice a week, with at least one day of rest in between sessions. Note that the exercises in this book are specific to your shoulders and aren't a substitute for strength training for other parts of your body.

14. Continue to monitor your ROM. As we noted in chapter 1, we all lose a certain amount of our flexibility as we age. There are a couple of strategies for minimizing this. One way would be to continue with your stretching exercises once a week to maintain your ROM level. Another idea would be to measure your ROM once per month, and If any decrease in ROM is detected, then return to doing the stretches on a daily basis until your desired ROM level has been re-established.

Appendixes

Appendix 1. Shoulder Anatomy

This appendix describes the main parts of your shoulder including five bones, four muscles with their tendons, one joint and a bursa

Bones of Right Shoulder Seen From the Rear

Your main shoulder joint is called the *glenohumeral joint* (GH). It is a ball and socket joint similar to the assembly in a car which allow the rear view mirror to swivel in all directions. However, your GH joint can move further than the mirror because its socket is rather shallow so that motion is less restricted. The bone forming the socket is the *scapula* (shoulder blade). The top part of the *humerus* (upper arm bone) forms the ball. Forming a top to the joint is the *acromion* which branches off from the scapula.

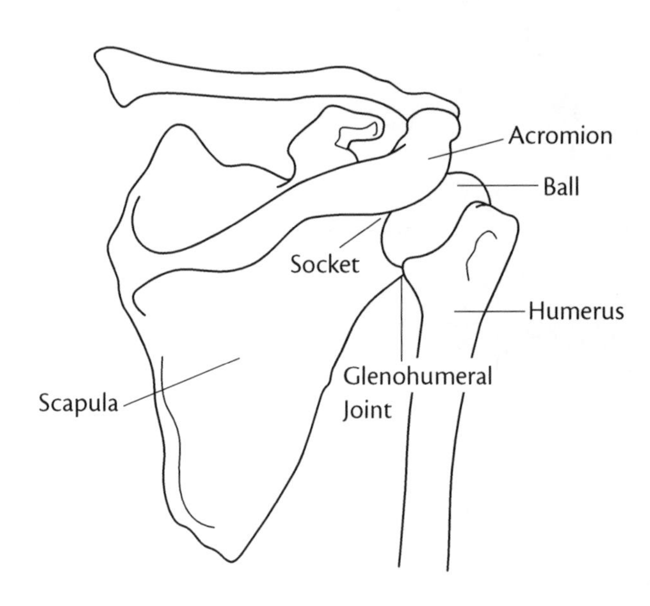

Bones of Right Shoulder Seen From the Front

The *clavicle* (collar bone) starts from a small joint at the *sternum*, the breast bone, in the center of your chest. The clavicle curves up and around your chest to meet up with the acromion at another small joint near the top of your shoulder.

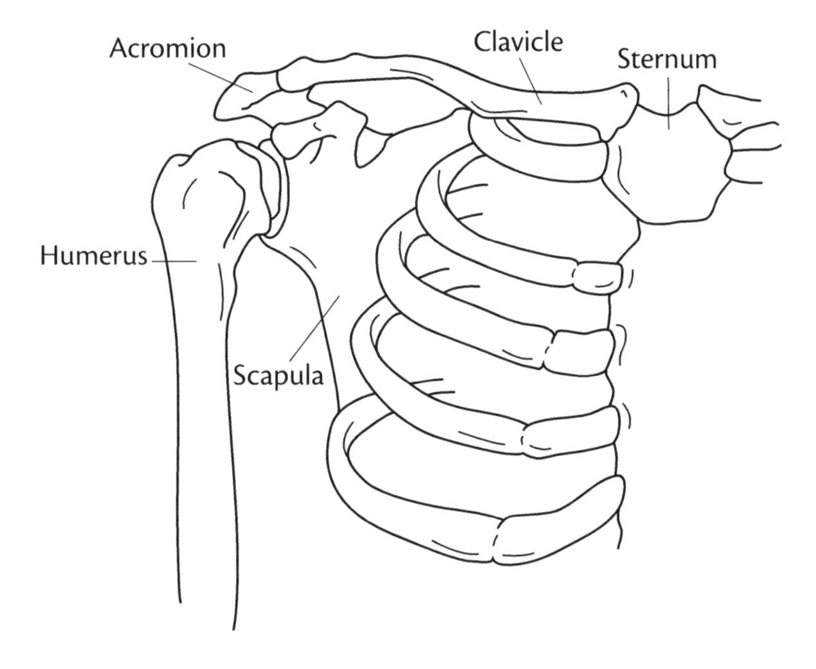

Muscles of Right Shoulder Seen From the Front

Your *rotator cuff* is a group of four tendons that encircle the ball of the humerus. Tendons are tissues which connect muscles to bone. Along with their associated muscles, they serve to keep your humerus firmly in its socket, as well as enable your arm to move in various ways. The rotator cuff muscles and tendons can be remembered by the acronym ***SITS***, for ***s****upraspinatus*, ***i****nfraspinatus*, ***t****eres minor,* and ***s****ubscapularis*.

Supraspinatus. Connects the top of the Scapula to the top of the Humerus. Allows sideways upward movement of the arm {Abduction).

Subscapularis. Attaches the whole front of the scapula to the humerus. Rotates the arm internally towards the body (Internal Rotation).

Just under the clavicle bone is another structure called a *bursa*, a fluid-filled sack that keeps the muscles from rubbing against the bone. If the rotator cuff become compressed, causing the bursa to be squeezed, then the humerus will be unable to rotate freely in its socket. This is called an *impingement*.

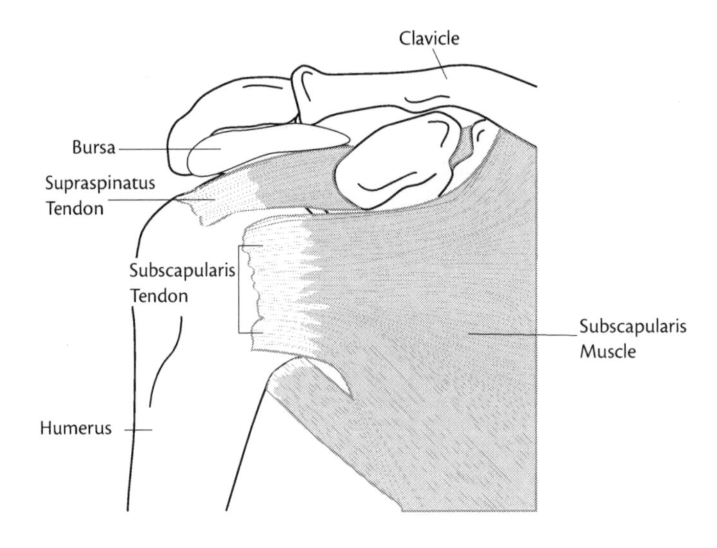

Muscles of Right Shoulder Seen From the Rear

The last two muscles and tendons are the

Infraspinatus. Connects from the back of the scapula to the humerus. It enables the arm to rotate away from the body (external rotation).

Teres minor. This muscle and tendon work in conjunction with the infraspinatus to enable external rotation. It lies below and alongside the infraspinatus.

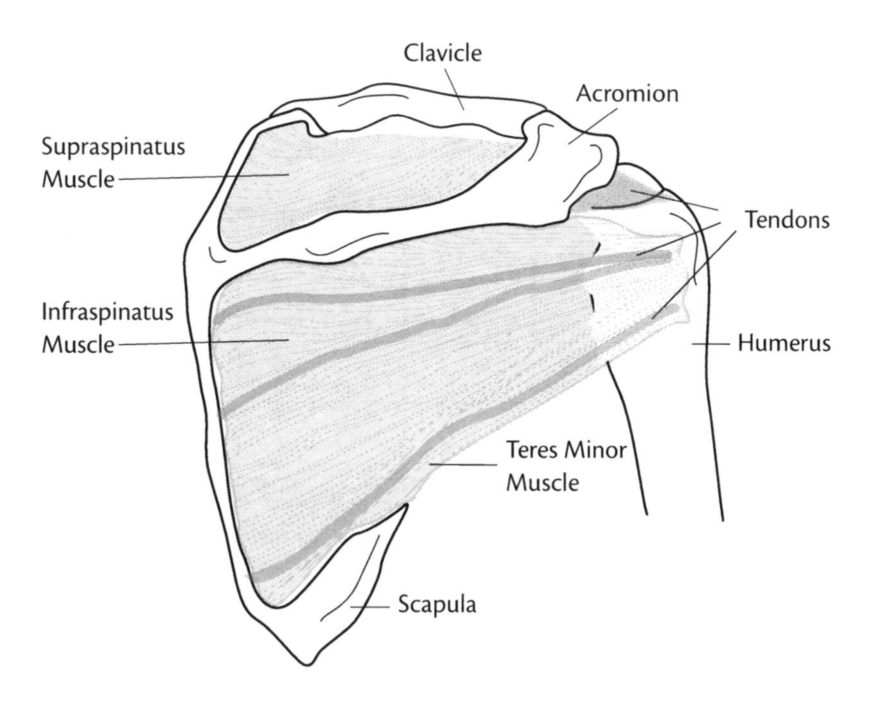

Appendix 2. Range of Motion Assessment

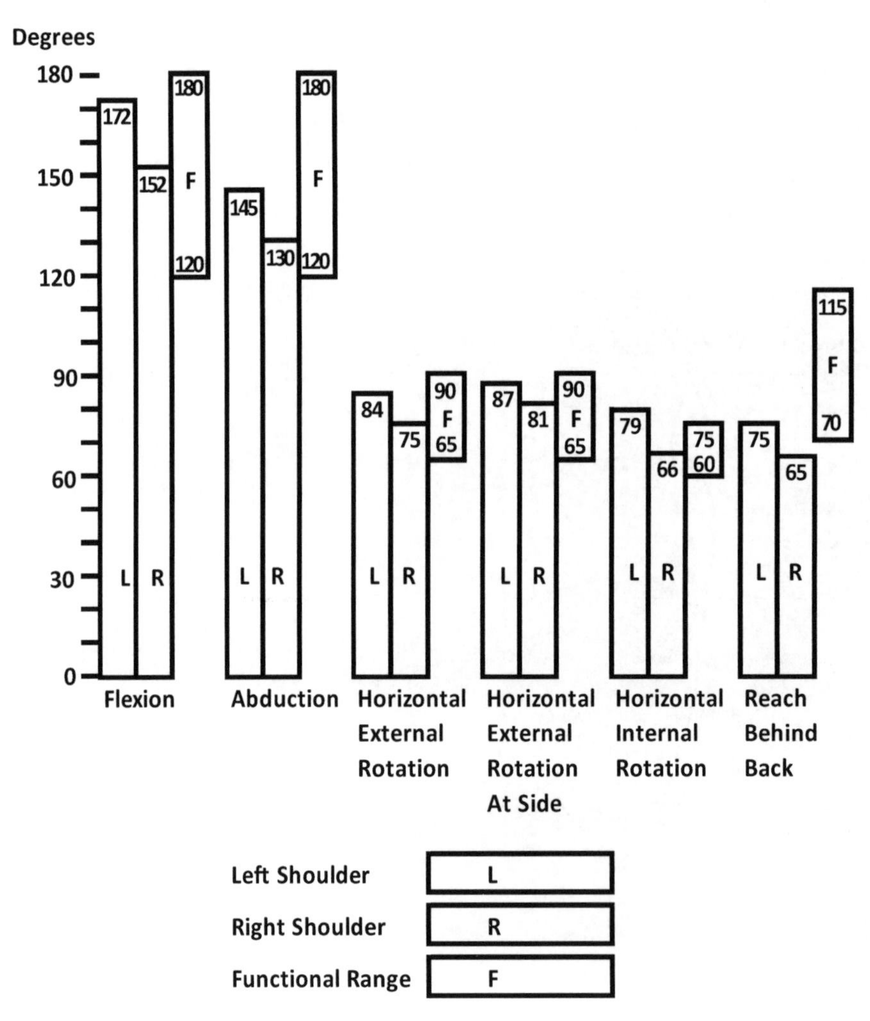

Graphed with Microsoft Excel

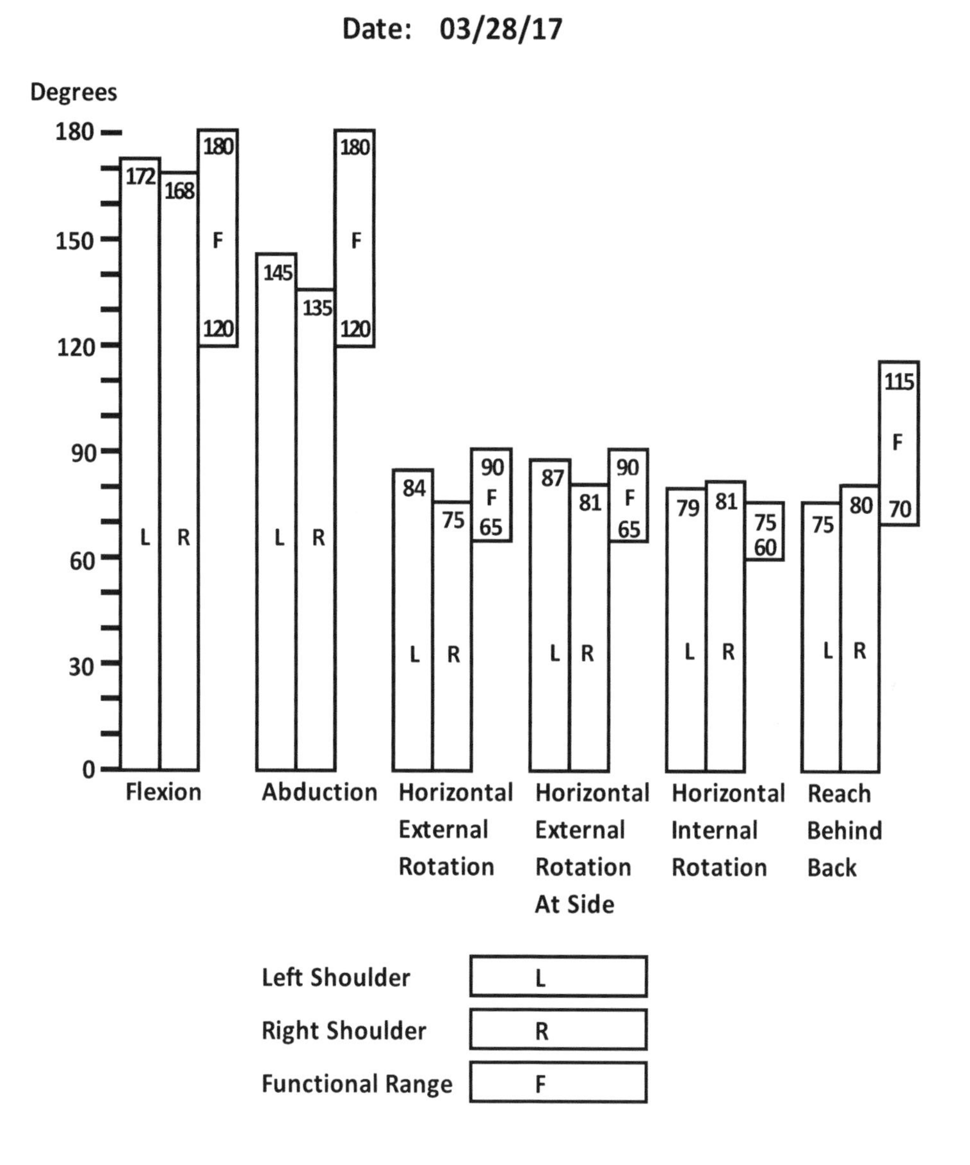

Graphed with Microsoft Excel

Appendix 3. Forecast Summary Sheet

STRETCHING	START	FINISH
STRENGTH TRAINING		
WIND DOWN/FINAL HEALING		

Appendix 4. Equipment Needed

Sources of Supply

Appendix 7, *Resources*, lists a number of suppliers. You can also discuss supplies with a physical therapist as they can recommend suppliers and sometimes they sell equipment as well. For traditional bricks-and-mortar shopping, your local drugstore and sporting goods store can supply some items. The Therapy Blocks and Therapy Straps used in our exercises can be purchased from us, or you can make them yourself or improvise. See below for more information.

Equipment

Cane
See "Stick."

Cold packs
See hot and cold packs.

Dumbbells
See "weights."

Hot and cold packs
Many of these products can be used for both hot and cold treatments, often by using a microwave to heat them up or a refrigerator to cool them down. However, it's often more convenient to have two products, one for hot and one for cold, which should be practical since these products aren't very expensive. For the heat treatments, a hot pack with *moist* heat is preferred. Since there is such a bewildering array of choices in these products, you might want to ask your practitioner or a pharmacist for a recommendation.

Towels. In order to apply heat, you can soak a towel in water, ring it out, and put it in the microwave for a minute or two. This has several advantages: it produces a very moist heat, the towel can be wrapped around the shoulder to be applied evenly where it's needed, and it's inexpensive. The downside is that the heat may not last very long and the towel would need to be reheated. Also, you may get wetter than you would like with this method. For cold treatments, a wet towel can be placed in a plastic bag and put in the freezer.

Hot/cold bags. For a cold treatment, you can put ice cubes in a plastic bag and put it on your shoulder. (With a suitable layer of cloth in between to protect your shoulder from ice burns.) A sack of frozen food such as peas also works. We recommend this option if you have a fresh injury and nothing else would be available quickly.

For a commercial solution, bags are available that have wide mouths that you can drop ice cubes into for icing the shoulder, as well as pour hot water into for heating the shoulder (just like with a hot water bottle). One disadvantage is that they may not wrap around your shoulder as much as you would like. It also may take a while to heat the water to put in the bag. These come in various sizes, such as 6, 9, and 11 inches in diameter. We have seen them advertised online for $13.

Gel packs. The hot and cold gel packs are convenient to heat in the microwave. To cool them, they are just stored in the freezer, ready for instant use. With their rectangular shape they can be wrapped around the shoulder, and they come in various sizes. On Amazon we have seen them range from five by ten inches for $6 to 11 by 14 inches for $11. One downside to these products is that the gel inside can be a fairly obnoxious chemical. If the container starts to leak, you may notice a very bad smell. Be on the lookout for this and replace the product promptly if it happens.

Log sheets

These are used to record the progress you are making in your stretching and strength training exercises. Samples can be found in Appendixes 5 and 6. You can also record your progress digitally on your PC, such as with an Excel worksheet.

Marking pen, fine point

This is used to record your progress on the Wall Reach stretching exercise.

Painter's tape or other masking tape

This has several uses:

- It can be put on the wall or door jamb to write on to record progress on the Wall Reach exercise.
- It can be wrapped around the cord of a pulley to record progress when doing pulley exercises.
- A couple of strips can be wrapped around the rod one is using for flexibility exercises "Standing Extension with Rod" and "Internal Rotation with Rod."

Pulley

We highly recommend shoulder pulleys—they provide a very effective passive shoulder stretch for the critical "reaching-up-above-the-head" movement. This kind of exercise is also one that can be measured quantitatively simply by wrapping a piece of tape around the cord to mark your spot, so we like it for that reason as well. It gives great satisfaction to move your tape up the cord each week as your range of motion improves.

We have seen around 15 different brands of these advertised online for around $7 to $33 dollars. It's not necessary to spend a lot of money on this, but get a sturdy one. Read the reviews or ask your practitioner for a recommendation. Your practitioner may even sell them.

The most critical consideration in using a pulley may be in deciding on a way to mount it. We prefer that it be mounted in such a way that you can lift your weak shoulder straight up with it; but if not, then just "up" will do. It's common to hook them to the top of a door. If you face the door when using the pulley then you couldn't make a 90 degree angle, but if your back is to the door, then you could. If you have access to exposed beams in a house, garage, carport, or pergola, they would make a very sturdy mounting platform, too. So might a tree limb.

When using your pulley, you will be putting a lot of tension on it so that if any component of the system should fail, the pulley could fly down and whack your head. If using a door, make sure that the door won't open by itself or that someone else might open it from the other side while you are exercising. If you leave your pulley outside, then sun and moisture will eventually weaken the cord to where it could break unexpectedly. Inspect the system every time you use it, be careful, and use common sense.

Resistance bands and tubing

There are a lot of trade-offs to consider when acquiring resistance bands, tubing, or weights to use with your strength training. This is a topic where a physical therapist could be very informative in helping you with your decision. Sometimes, though, they just give or sell you a particular product without going into detail about all of the options that are out there. We hope that the following discussion will help make you a more knowledgeable consumer and also give you some things to talk about if you do go over it with your practitioner.

All of the strength training exercises that we do with weights can also be done with elastic exercise bands or tubes.

Some advantages of bands and tubes are that

- They are lightweight so that you can take them with you if you travel
- They can provide resistance in the horizontal plane, not just the vertical, so a great number of exercises are possible

Some advantages of weights are that

- They last forever
- The amount of resistance that you are using can be measured very precisely

A longer discussion of this topic can be found online at

https://bodylastics.com/elastic-resistance-vs-free-weights-by-jim-stoppani-phd/

If you do decide to go with elastic resistance material, you then need to decide which kind, bands or tubing? Resistance *bands* are typically five feet long and four inches wide, and may be made from latex or some other material. Resistance *tubing* typically runs from about 3-1/2 feet to four feet long, not including any handle, and is about 1/4 inch in diameter. Both types of equipment come in different resistance levels, which are color coded, generally with lighter colors providing the least resistance and darker colors the most.

If you happen to be allergic to latex, then you may need to find a product with no latex in it. If you're not using a handle, then the bands may be more comfortable to grasp since they are wider. There is a different feel to it when using bands or tubing, so you may have a preference for one over the other. Finally, there is a safety issue in that bands and tubes will eventually wear out. You don't want your band to suddenly snap and jerk your arm. There are several ways to reduce the danger of your equipment breaking:

- Don't over stretch the material. Consult the manufacturer or your practitioner about what is a safe range for stretching it.
- Some tubing comes with a fabric cord inside of it which prevents the user from stretching the tube to where it's likely to break. If it were to break, the cord would help to suppress any uncontrolled snap. One brand with this feature is called "Bodylastics," (see bodylastics.com).
- If you are going to use bands to stay in shape for life, then consider replacing them periodically, such as every year, even if it comes with a lifetime warranty. Again, you might want to consult with the manufacturer or your practitioner. The following link discusses this topic in greater detail:

https://bodylastics.com/blog/secret-to-prevent-resistance-bands-snapping/

There are also some common extras that people use with their bands such as handles, fasteners for doors and other anchors, and loops to put their feet in. It might be more economical in the long run to buy a set that includes several bands or tubes with different resistance levels as well as a variety of attachments. We have seen a 12-piece set advertised online for $30 which should be more than adequate for shoulder rehabilitation.

Rod
See "stick."

Ruler or tape measure

This is useful in the "Wall Reach" exercise to mark off 1/4-inch increments for stretching. If you are using a stack of books and magazines to measure your stretches in our four core stretching exercises, it can be used to quantify those measurements. It may also be used with pulley exercises to mark off your stretching distances there, too.

Stick

A whole class of stretching exercises uses some sort of "stick" as an aid. It could be a yardstick, cane, ski pole, a dowel rod, a handle from a plumber's helper, a curtain rod, or even a long cardboard tube that rolls of paper come on. You could use different pieces of equipment for different exercises if they worked better for you. In general, we like something that is two to three feet long, lightweight, and has a hook or knob on one end that can be grasped by the weak hand. After doing a static stretch, we find it less of a strain to grasp the rod with our weak hand and let our well arm pull our weak arm back to the neutral position. We find that a 28 inch telescoping projection rod is good for this. These are the white rods with a 90-degree bend at each end that are often used to hang curtains on bathroom windows. They are fairly inexpensive; they can be found for around $2 as we write this.

Therapy Blocks

These are used in four of our key stretching exercises to measure the distance of the stretch and also provide a platform to stretch against. These can be improvised for free or for little cost, or they can be purchased from us under the "ROMdoc™" trademark.

1. Improvise

A stack of books and magazines are ready-made blocks that can be used to perform the stretching exercises. For example, Phone books and National Geographic magazines work quite well. You can stack up the materials and measure the height with a tape measure, or you can directly record the number of books/magazines used for each exercise and use that as your measuring method.

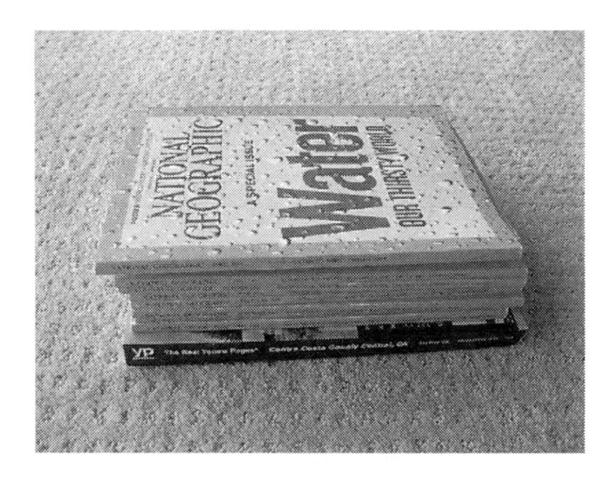

National Geographic Magazines
and a phone book

2. Ready-made therapy blocks.

For the convenience of our readers, we offer these blocks for sale on eBay. To find them, simply key in the word "ROMdoc" in the search box. That is our trademark, which stands for "Range of Motion Doctor." Both the "ROMdoc™ therapy blocks" and "ROMdoc™ therapy straps" should appear.

We provide the blocks in sets of eight (8) pieces which can be stacked from 1/4 inch up to 17-3/4 inches in height. The blocks are roughly 10-1/2 inches in length by 8-1/2 inches in width, and heights vary from 1/4 inch up to six inches. Shown In the picture below, from left to right, are two 6-inch blocks, one 3-inch block, two 1-inch blocks, and three pieces in front that are 1/4 inch thick.

The blocks are made out of cardboard and assembly is required, which should take around one and a half hours, on average. Shipping tape and glue are needed to put the blocks together. Anyone with the ability to wrap packages and prepare them for mailing should be able to assemble these blocks. Prices may vary, of course, but as of the first edition of this book, in 2018, we anticipate that the price will be around $76 including shipping.

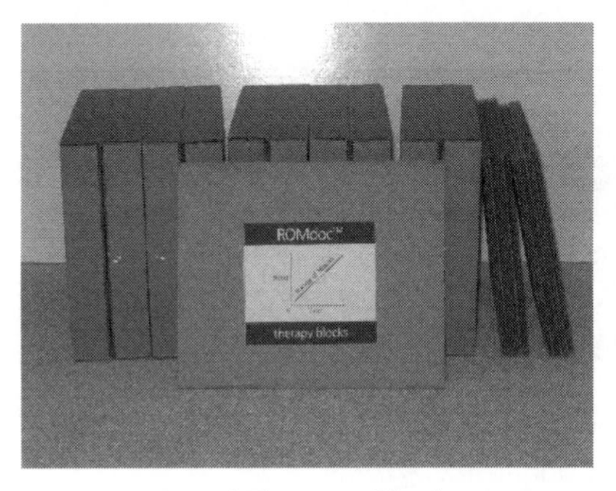

Set of Therapy Blocks

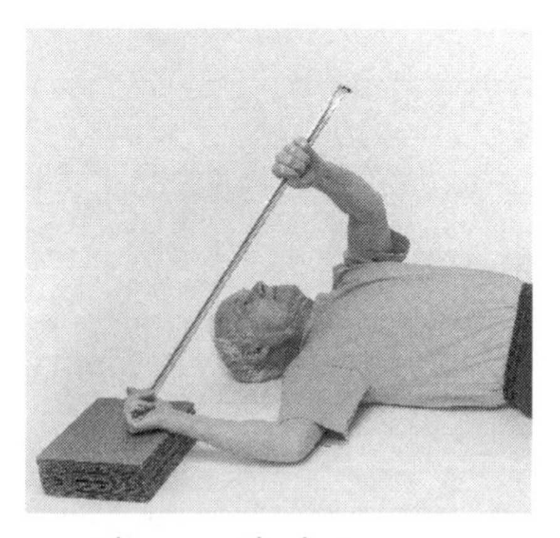

Therapy Blocks in use

Therapy Straps

These are used for two of our stretching exercises, "Abduction" and "Internal Rotation behind the Back." These can be made by hand, or they can be purchased pre-made.

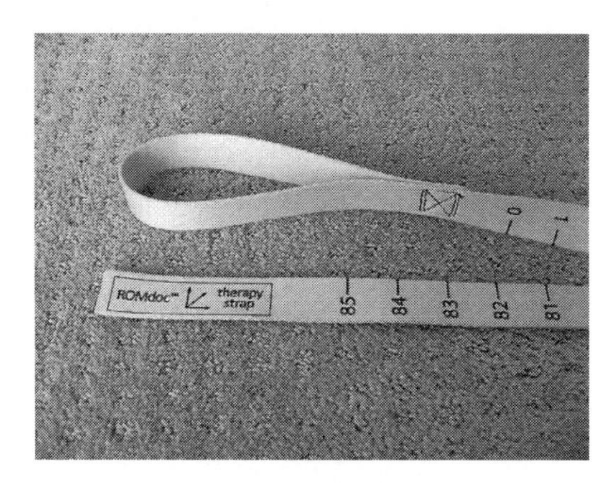

Commercial Therapy Strap

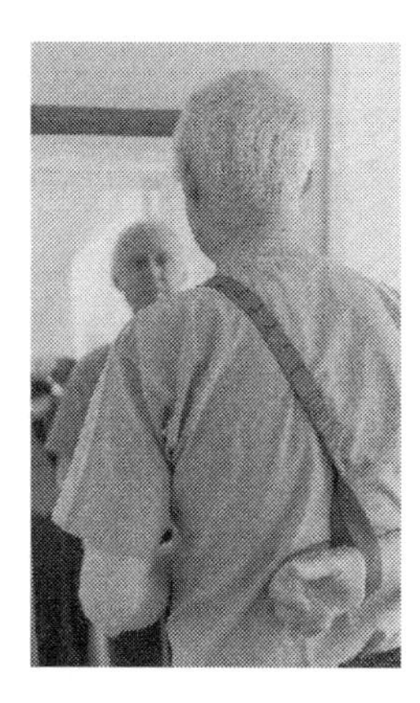

"Reach behind the Back" using strap

Making Your Own Therapy Straps

These can be made from 8-foot yoga straps which are readily available from retailers for under $10. Many have a D-ring at one end which is used to make a loop. Just make sure that the loop doesn't slip at all as that could throw off the measurements. Tape the strap down straight on a hard surface and lay a tape measure beside it. Then, using a fine-point marking pen, draw lines at one inch intervals as shown in the picture above and you're ready to go.

Commercial Therapy Straps

At the time of this writing, we are currently offering pre-made straps on eBay under the trademark "ROMdoc™ therapy straps." The price is around $28 postpaid. Simply key in "ROMdoc" in the search box on eBay.

Weights

You could use elastic bands instead of weights for your strength training so you might want to give this some thought. See our discussion under "elastic bands and tubes" and talk to your practitioner about what would work best for you.

Weights can be classified as weight machines and free weights. Free weight types include dumbbells, barbells, medicine balls, sandbells, and kettlebells. For physical therapy of the shoulder, dumbbells are usually employed in a weight range of one to ten pounds. If your frame of reference is body building, then you might be surprised at the small amount of weight used here. We only recommend using weights up to four percent of body weight as we're working on small muscles here, besides which we want to avoid aggravating your shoulder injury.

Dumbbells can be purchased online or in stores. Amazon sells a set of two weights each, from one to five pound, from "CanDo" for under $60. That doesn't include tax and shipping. Another nice-to-have might be a rack to store them on which could run another $25 or so. If you need more weights, such as from six to ten pounds, they can be purchased individually or as sets as well.

Appendix 5. Stretching Log Form

Exercise:								
Left					Right			
Degrees	Inches	Reps	Time		Degrees	Inches	Reps	Time

Appendix 6. Strength Training Log Form

Date	Weight	Sets	Reps		Date	Weight	Sets	Reps
Internal Rotation					Internal Rotation			
Standing Low Row					Standing Low Row			
Scaption					Scaption			
External Rotation					External Rotation			
Side Lying Abduction					Side Lying Abduction			
Seated Horizontal Ext Rotation					Seated Horizontal Ext Rotation			
Standing Diagonal Raise					Standing Diagonal Raise			

Form for other exercises:

Date	Weight	Sets	Reps		Date	Weight	Sets	Reps

Appendix 7. Selected Resources

There are a lot of good suppliers and information sources that can be accessed on the internet. There are also a few of dubious value and perhaps even outright fraud. If something you see online sounds too good to be true, we suggest you get a second opinion from your health care provider(s) before entrusting your money, time, and well-being to an unverified site. Following are a few sites that we have found to be of interest.

Note that our listing here of these providers does not imply that we guarantee or endorse their products, the accuracy of their information, or the suitability of their products for your particular situation.

Amazon
www.amazon.com

They sell resistance bands, tubing, dumbbells, shoulder pulleys, physical therapy books, projection curtain rods (for exercises requiring a stick, cane, or rod), and goniometers (instruments for measuring range of motion). If you like shopping at Amazon, then it's certainly worth a look here.

American Association of Orthopedic Surgeons
http://orthoinfo.org/PDFs/Rehab_Shoulder_5.pdf

This site provide a ten-page document with stretching and strengthening exercises for the shoulder which can be viewed online or downloaded. It also has many other instruction sheets, articles, and videos covering a wide array of orthopedic topics.

Bodylastics
Bodylastics.com
561-562-4745
These folks sell a variety of elastic exercise bands and tubes. They also have some free information that you can browse through. Click on "blog" in the upper right-hand corner of the page or scroll way down to the bottom and peruse the articles found there. Here are a few samples that you might find interesting:

https://bodylastics.com/elastic-resistance-vs-free-weights-by-jim-stoppani-phd/

https://bodylastics.com/blog/4-must-do-rotator-cuff-exercises-with-exercise-bands/

https://bodylastics.com/blog/secret-to-prevent-resistance-bands-snapping/

Google
www.google.com
Of course, a Google search is a good place to start to find a huge selection of references to a wide range of topics. For example, a Google search can be used to find instructions on how to use a goniometer to measure shoulder ROM. Just key in "how to use a goniometer to measure shoulder flexion" and the following excellent You Tube video will be presented:

https://www.youtube.com/watch?v=3CcnTvkjI_0

Mayo Foundation for Medical Education and Research
http://www.mayoclinic.org/
They provide free, authoritative information on a wide variety of health topics. You can search the site using the "Search Mayo Clinic" search bar at the top, or use the "Patient Care & Health Info" tab where you can look up symptoms, diseases, tests, and drugs alphabetically. For example, good instructions for proper posture can be found here:

http://www.mayoclinic.org/healthy-lifestyle/adult-health/multimedia/back-pain/sls-20076817?s=5

North Coast Medical Inc.
www.ncmedical.com
800-821-9319
This site is geared more towards professionals, but it's an interesting site for browsing. They have an in-house team of physical and occupational therapists, so if you have questions about suitable products, this should be a good source. You can phone or chat online with them. It's also a good place to find more specialized items such as goniometers.

Physical Therapy Clinics
Sometimes your own physical therapist may have products available in her shop, but may overlook telling you about it. Do feel free to ask your therapist if you can buy products from her clinic and/or discuss equipment and where to buy it.

Pro Therapy Supplies
www.protherapysupplies.com
1-800-883-0368
This company carries the most commonly used products for shoulder therapy: dumbbells, exercise bands and tubes, hot and cold packs, and shoulder pulleys. They also sell goniometers.

Rehab Mart
www.rehabmart.com
1-800-827-8283
This company sells a wide variety of physical therapy equipment. Tabs on the website enable customers to view products by category, brand, and body part. For example, you can drill down by "body part/shoulder." Other searches by "category/range of motion therapy" and "category/range of motion instruments" are also useful. Some of the sections also have interesting articles such as this article on range of motion:

https://www.rehabmart.com/category/range_of_motion_therapy.htm#bottom

At the bottom of the website there are various interesting links. Under PT Show you can schedule a session with a physical therapist remotely over the internet!

Theraband
www.theraband.com
1-800-321-2135

These folks invented elastic exercise bands some 40 years ago. In addition to their products, they provide some interesting free information. Click on the "Resources" tab at the top and check out the material on "research" and "care and safety."

WebMD, LLC.
www.webmd.com

Look up health topics from A to Z, get information on drugs, healthy living advice, and more.

Endnotes

1. Knopf, 25.

2. Sharecare, Inc. "Will I lose flexibility as I age?" Accessed May 10, 2017. https://www.sharecare.com/health/aging-and-fitness/lose-flexibility-age

3. Mayo Foundation for Medical Education and Research. "Fitness training: Elements of a well-rounded routine." Accessed May 10, 2017. http://www.mayoclinic.org/healthy-lifestyle/fitness/in-depth/fitness-training/art-20044792?pg=1

4. Buffalo Rehab Group Physical Therapy. "Three Reasons Posture Is Causing Your Shoulder Pain." Accessed June 21, 2017. http://buffalorehab.com/blog/3-ways-bad-posture-hurting-shoulder/

5. WebMD, LLC. "7 Wonders of Water." Accessed May 13, 2017. http://www.webmd.com/diet/ss/slideshow-water-health

6. Mayo Foundation for Medical Education and Research. "Aerobic exercise: Top 10 reasons to get physical." Accessed May 13, 2017. http://www.mayoclinic.org/healthy-lifestyle/fitness/in-depth/aerobic-exercise/art-20045541?pg=1

7. Knopf, 25.

8. Schiff, xiii.

9. Same as note number 4.

10. Knopf, 25.
Knopf writes "Note that the absence of symptoms does not mean full restoration."

11. Same as note number 8.

Works Cited

American Association of Orthopedic Surgeons
http://orthoinfo.org/PDFs/Rehab_Shoulder_5.pdf

Buffalo Rehab Group Physical Therapy.
http://buffalorehab.com

Knopf, Dr. Karl. *Healthy Shoulder Handbook*. Berkeley, CA: Ulysses Press, 2010.

Mayo Foundation for Medical Education and Research
http://www.mayoclinic.org/

Schiff, Brian, PT, CSCS. *The Ultimate Frozen Shoulder Therapy Guide*. B Fit Training Systems, LLC.

Sharecare, Inc.
https://www.sharecare.com/health/aging-and-fitness/lose-flexibility-age

WebMD, LLC.

Index

I

L

M

N

P

R

S

T

W

Y

About the Author

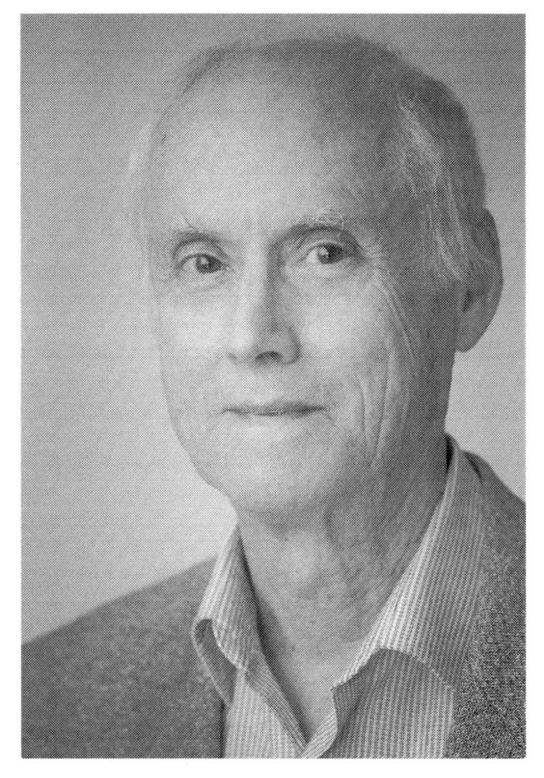

Melvin Rosenthal

Melvin graduated from the University of California at Berkeley in 1968 with a BA degree in math. He worked in the software field for 33 years as a programmer, systems analyst, supervisor, researcher and writer. When he suffered a frozen shoulder, he put his analytical skills to work to enhance the standard stretching exercises to make them as effective as possible. This book is the result.

Made in the USA
Middletown, DE
13 April 2019